Walking

Nature's Perfect Exercise

by Pamela Kihm

Illustrations by Sharron Ott

ISBN 0-9779102-2-9

Second printing
Production: Matthew Doherty
Print Editors: May Ruth Spitzer, Donnelly Barclay
Artistic Editor: Sharron Ott
Illustrations: Sharron Ott

Published by
PainFreeChoices® Evanston, Illinois
Web: http://www.painfreechoices.com

Dedicated to you, the reader...

Those of you about to tackle days of walking to raise funds for cancer research (or any other health research) have my endless admiration and are my inspiration for *Walking: Nature's Perfect Exercise* to be in print by Springtime.

Within these pages you'll find guidance and experiments, as well as exercises, to help you walk more efficiently — whether to simply cross the street or to hike trails. The format is in "STEPS," a practical pun — i.e. don't skip over any of the STEPS.

May this book help your every step lead to better quality of life.

Pamela Kihm

Books by Pamela Kihm

Stop Sciatica Now:
Help Yourself Eliminate Back and Leg Pain

Relax Your Back With a Roller:
Exercises and Strategies to Eliminate Pain

Walking: Nature's Perfect Exercise

Ms Kihm's Website:
www.painfreechoices.com

Table of Contents

FIRST STEP...
Allow the Front of You to Lengthen

There is a definite relationship between your posture and the degree of ease you'll have while walking. You already know that. However, you may not be aware that some of your efforts to maintain your posture may actually be making walking more difficult.

The way you maintain your posture may be challenging your ability to walk comfortably and powerfully.

How do you gain posture that's upright? Do you pull your shoulders back? What do you do to maintain upright posture?

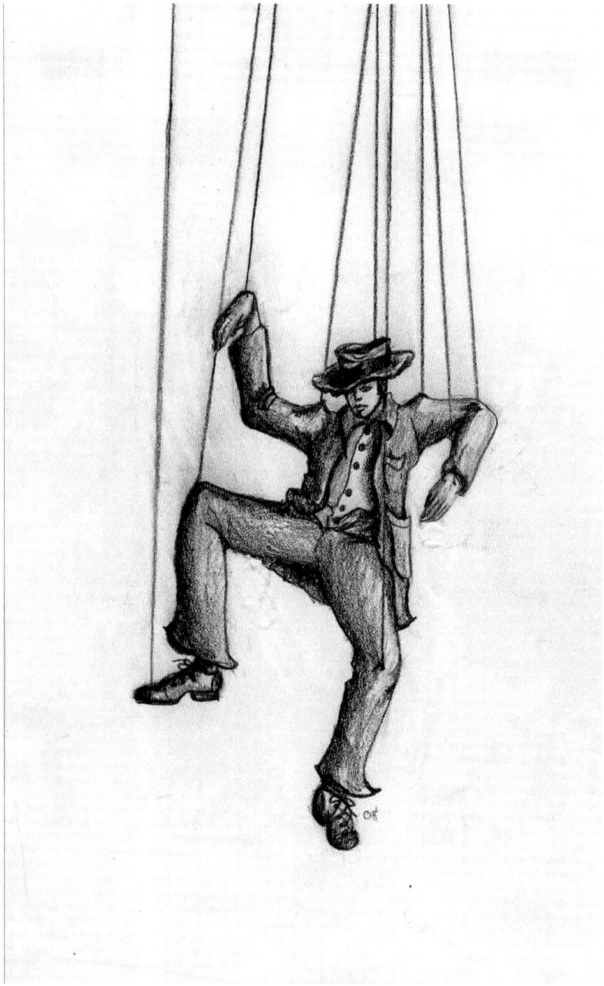

Any of those three might work long-term if we humans were marionettes with strings holding us up.

EXPERIMENT...
Posture from the Top Down?

1. Stand resting both hands on the top of the back of a sturdy chair or have your hands rest on a table top or countertop.
2. Slouch. Then, as if you're seven years old and your teacher commands, "stand up straight," improve your posture.
3. Slouch again so you can discover what you actually do to bring yourself upright out of a slouch...

   Do you pull your head up? If so, does the rest of your body follow?

   Do you pull your shoulders back? If so, does that cause tension in your upper back and does your head remain forward in spite of pulling your shoulders back?

   Do you pull your chest up? If so, how does this affect your breathing? Could you stay this way for very long?

Since you are not a marionette, would you like to learn how to maintain posture from the bottom up?

Exercise One... Posture from the Bottom Up

1. Sit on a firm chair without your back touching the chair.
2. Position your feet a comfortable distance apart, making firm contact with the ground. Allow your knees to be as wide apart as the distance between your two feet.
3. Place both hands at your waist with your thumbs forward and your fingertips to the left and the right of your sacrum (five fused vertebrae in the center back of your pelvic bowl).
4. Slouch and notice that the top of your sacrum — your whole pelvic bowl — tilts backward a bit.
5. Rearrange your pelvis so that the top of your sacrum is no longer tilted backward.

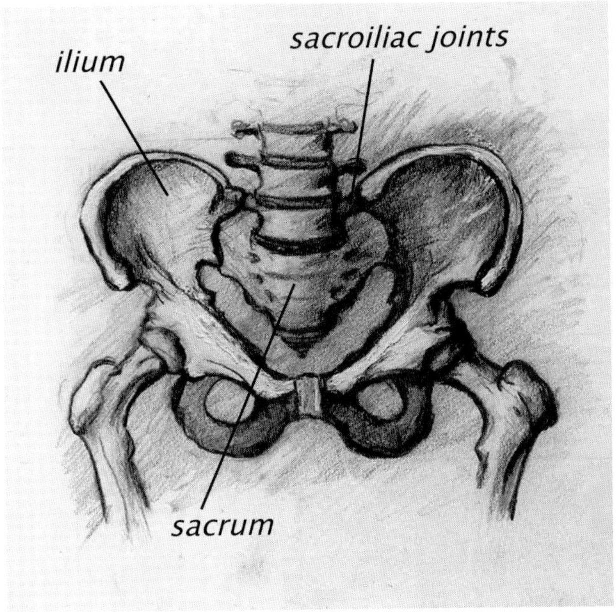

Your pelvic bowl contains the base of your spine — the five fused vertebrae of your sacrum which is connected to each ilium (hip bone) through your sacroiliac joints ("SI joints").

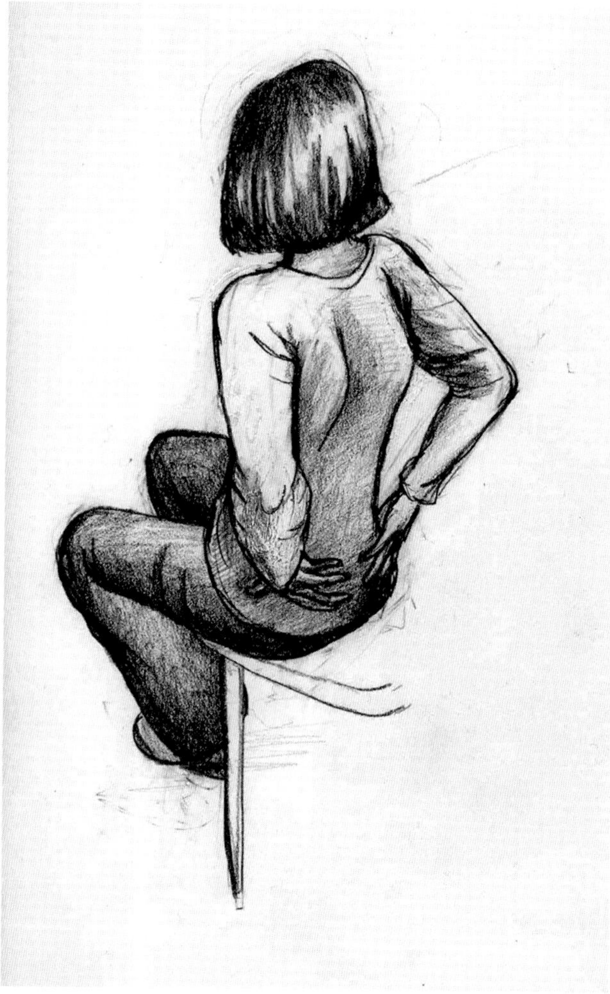

6. Gently do this combination of slouching and then rearranging your pelvis a few times.

   Notice that each time you rearrange your pelvis so that your sacrum is vertical instead of tilted — you are no longer slouched.

   Your pelvic bowl has a powerful influence on your posture.

7. As you rest for a moment think about how your spine is the connecting link between your pelvis and your skull, and that your ribs wrap around from your spine to your sternum ("breastbone").

8. Place the palm of one hand on your sternum in the center front of your chest, and the back of the other hand on your sacrum in the center back of your pelvis.

9. Sink your sternum a little bit and notice that no matter how little you sink your sternum, the top of your sacrum correspondently tilts backward.

10. Notice that each time your pelvis rearranges to un-tilt your sacrum, your sternum is passively lifted and the front of you lengthens.

    Notice if it's easier to breathe fully when the front of you is lengthened.

11. Stand behind the chair with your hands resting on the top of the back of the chair.

12. Let your sternum sink and notice that no matter how little you sink your sternum, your coccyx ("tailbone") at the bottom of your sacrum scoops forward and under you.

    Rearrange your pelvis so that your coccyx is no longer scooped under you and your sacrum is more perpendicular to the ground.

    Consequently, your sternum also comes up to be perpendicular to the ground — and the front of you lengthens!

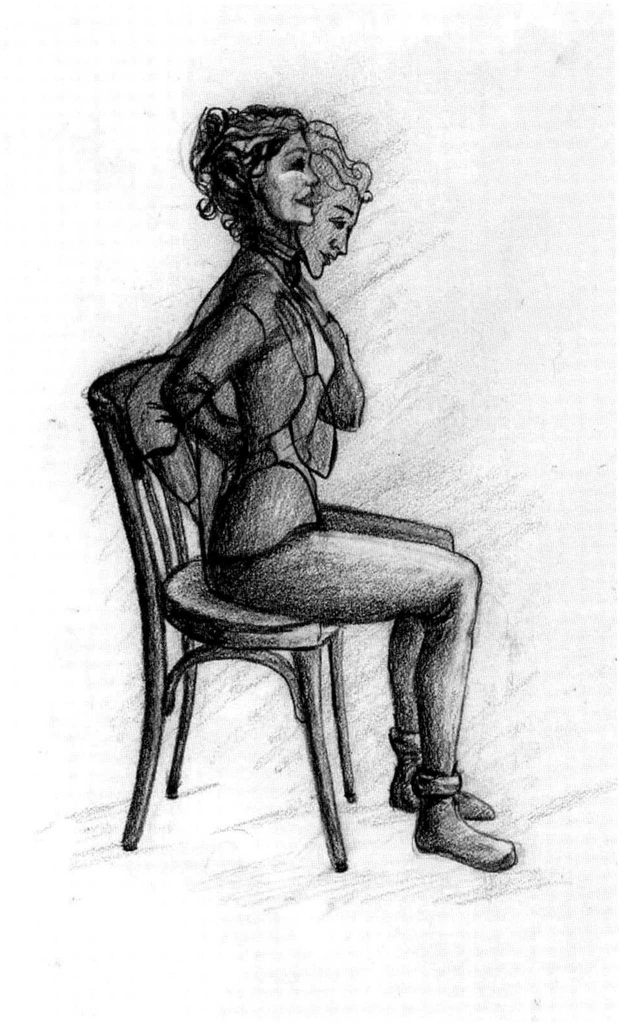

When your sternum and your sacrum are perpendicular to the ground, your whole spine is supported by your pelvis.

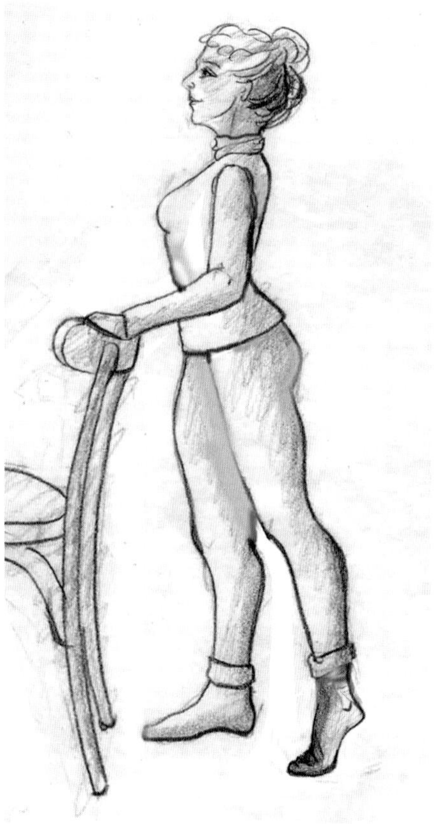

EXERCISE TWO... Encouraging Upright Lengthening

1. Stand facing a countertop or the back of a sturdy chair, close enough that your elbows are bent when you rest your hands on that surface.
2. Place your feet directly under your body as if they're on parallel tracks, with the space between your feet a bit less than the distance between your shoulders.
3. Slide one foot back — "on those parallel tracks" — far enough back so the toes of that foot are parallel with the heel of your front foot.
4. Allow the heel of the foot that is behind you to peel off the ground. (Leave your toes and the "ball" of that foot on the ground.)

   Allow the front of that ankle to lengthen to make it even easier for your heel to peel off the ground.
5. Do #4 several times slowly, allowing the front of your body to lengthen each time your back heel peels off the ground.

Your toes and the ball of the foot that is behind remain in constant contact with the ground.

Don't tighten muscles in the front or the back of your torso — just think skeletally.

6. Switch the position of your feet so that your other foot can take a turn behind you with that heel peeling away from the ground.

   Each time the heel of this foot (that is now behind you) peels off the ground, allow the front of you to "get tall."

   Your foot that is in front remains in place, making full contact with the ground. Your toes and the ball of the foot that is behind also remain in full contact with the ground until step #7.

7. Now walk across the room or down the hall with each heel taking its turn to peel off the ground.

As each heel takes its turn to peel off the ground, allow the lengthening through the front of your ankle to be echoed in lengthening through the front of your body.

Slouching is just one of the many possible ways to crunch the front of you. Since your spine is a continuum from the bottom of your coccyx (tailbone) to the top of your neck, any one of the following can compromise your walking as well as your comfort and your breathing:

- ⃠ Looking at your feet so that your 12–15 pound head hangs forward;
- ⃠ Intentionally tucking your coccyx forward and under you;
- ⃠ Tightening through your gluteal (buttocks) muscles — which rearranges the position of your pelvis and your spine, resulting in the tucking of your coccyx;
- ⃠ Tightening through your lower back flattens away your lumbar curve (gentle curve nature intended for your lower back) — which results in subtly tilting your sacrum so that the bottom of your sacrum and your coccyx move forward and under you.

Whether exercising (or just moving through your day) you can create lower back problems if you try to protect your lumbar vertebrae by constantly tightening through your lower back.

Unfortunately there are countless books and articles available that advise you to "tighten your abs" and/or "tighten your gluts" as you walk. Try the following experiment to discover for yourself if that's really in your best interest.

EXPERIMENT...

To Crunch or Not to Crunch While Walking

1. Walk down the hall with your "gluts" held tightly.

   Can you walk with your gluts held tightly without your thigh muscles tensing?

2. Stop and wiggle out any tension in your body.
3. Now walk down the hall with your gluts relaxed, allowing your pelvis to support your posture, simply thinking skeletally. (See page 5)
4. Alternate between #1 and #3 to see which way helps and which way interferes with your walking.
5. Now walk down the hall with your "abs" held tightly.

Habitual ways of standing and walking, although very familiar, may not be functional.

Can you walk this way without your lower back and pelvis being rearranged in such a way that your coccyx tucks under?

6. Stop and wiggle out any tension in your body.
7. Now walk down the hall with your abs neutral, simply skeletally allowing your pelvis to lengthen the front of you instead of crunching the front of you.
8. Alternate between #5 and #7 to see which way helps and which way interferes with your walking.

Dr. Moshe Feldenkrais (1904–1984), the originator of the Feldenkrais Method® of Somatic Education upon which this book is based, taught people a simple trick to gain "good posture." He said, "Pretend that you are about to jump upward."

Any changes in body positioning that enabled each person to be in the position as if to jump upward was exactly what each individual needed for *functional upright posture,* i.e. ready to move without having to rearrange one's body or the way the feet are positioned.

EXPERIMENT…

Clever Technique to Gain Upright Posture

1. Stand where you have some room to move.
2. Notice anything in particular about the way you are standing that might be counterproductive to taking that first step if you were going to walk across the room.
3. Experiment by pretending to jump straight upward. **(It's important to test that this theory works without actually jumping, just imagining that you're about to jump upward.)**
4. Notice what you do to rearrange your body as you imagine yourself preparing to jump upward.
5. Relax while standing.
6. Again, pretend that you're going to jump upward so you can really pay attention to where you make subtle changes in your body positioning:
   - ~ Did you allow more bend-ability through your hip joints and knees?

Some of our habits that give the illusion of being necessary for stability are exactly what we need to release in order to walk easily.

~ Did you rearrange the position of your back, shoulders, or head?

~ Did you shift your weight to be more centered?

~ Did you have to relax your abdominal muscles a bit?

~ Did you relax along your coccyx ("tailbone")?

~ Did you relax your toes?

Each change in your body positioning that makes it possible for you to "pretend to jump upward" is exactly what you need to be ready to walk comfortably and efficiently.

"We make the impossible possible, the possible easy, and the easy elegant."

— Moshe Feldenkrais

SECOND STEP...
Walk Smarter, Not Harder

There's a major misconception flourishing that walking is all about getting one foot out in front of the other. In fact, for "Gait Analysis" in the medical community the penultimate measure is how far each foot travels ahead of the other foot while walking.

The following is one of the biggest shifts in paradigm that will come from the reading of this book: Stepping far ahead of oneself is a waste of energy, even counterproductive. Why? It is the foot that is taking its turn behind you that propels you forward!

This shift, from tunnel vision on each foot as it takes its turn forward to focusing on each foot as it takes its turn behind you, is paramount!

EXPERIMENT…

Can the Foot that is Behind You Power You Forward?

1. Stand facing a countertop or tabletop with your hands lightly resting on that surface.
2. Place your feet directly under your body as if they are on parallel tracks with a space between your feet (and "the tracks") that is a bit less than the distance between your shoulders.
3. Slide your right foot back — on its "track" — far enough back so the toes of your right foot are parallel with the heel of your left foot.
4. Allow the heel of your right foot to peel off the ground slowly several times, with your toes and the "ball" of your right foot remaining in contact wth the ground.
5. Notice what happens with the rest of your body each time your right heel peels off the ground:

   Is your body gently propelled forward each time the heel of the foot that is behind you leaves the ground?

   Does it take any muscular effort through your torso for your body to move forward each time the heel of the foot that is behind you leaves the ground?

6. With your feet remaining in place as in #3 (your right foot back) have your left foot draw you forward.

   How much muscular effort does this take?

7. Alternate between having your front (left) foot draw your body forward and having your back (right) heel peel off the ground to move your body forward.

   Notice which way of moving your body forward takes less effort.

   Notice which way is more comfortable.

8. Switch your feet so that your right foot is forward and your left foot back and do #7.

9. Walk down the hall, noticing if there is a difference in your ease of walking if you have each foot (as it takes its turn in front of you) draw your body forward *or* having each foot (as it takes its turn behind you) propel you forward.

Does this help you understand why running competitors start a race by pushing off with whichever foot is behind instead of by reaching forward with the front foot?

Walking with your stride behind you encourages the front of you to lengthen, creating better posture and eliminating the need to strain through your back.

Striding out ahead is purely cultural, i.e. learned by copying others and thinking, "That's the way to get ahead in this world."

People who carry loads of lumber or jugs of water on top of their heads do not step out ahead of themselves. If they stepped out ahead, the jug of water or lumber would slip off — unless their muscles tensed to the point of pain and fatigue to compensate for lack of skeletal support from underneath. Instead, they allow each foot to take its turn landing right underneath them. As the heel of one foot finishes peeling off the ground behind them, the other foot is giving full support directly underneath the body. That is what propels them smoothly forward with comfort and strength.

When your stride is behind you, the heel of the foot that is taking its turn to land directly underneath you does make contact with the ground before the front of that foot. However, that moment when each heel first makes contact with the ground is just a split-second before your whole foot provides support.

At the beginning of the one mile, all-uphill hike out of the Grand Canyon after an incredible rafting trip, the raft-man directing us up Bright Angel Trail told us to "take little steps." I took his advice and the trek up was relatively easy in spite of the heat. I thought the excellent result was because I just wasn't "pushing myself," but I never forgot what he said.

Now more than twenty years later, seventeen of those years as a Feldenkrais® Practitioner, I'm well aware that by taking those "little steps" I was gaining twice the propulsion! If I had stepped out far ahead of myself, like my two teenagers, I would have missed half of the number of "push-offs" available to propel me forward — the push off from each foot as each heel peeled off the ground behind me.

Propelling yourself forward — instead of drawing yourself forward — is powerful!

You don't need to restrict yourself to little steps in order to have your stride behind you. Just don't step way out ahead! Simply let each foot in turn land right underneath you and — especially if you allow flexibility through your feet and ankles — your stride will gradually lengthen behind you.

"Stride" is simply the (forward/ backward) distance between your two feet as you walk. Having your stride behind you, instead of out in front of you, has many advantages:

- More efficient for more power
- More comfortable for your neck, back, hips, knees, and feet
- Not as likely to get heel spurs and heel calluses
- Encourages healthful posture
- Knees not as likely to hyperextend (knees so "straight" they actually bend a bit backward)

You don't need to work hard for your body to be propelled forward by each heel taking its turn to peel off the ground — just let it happen!

You might as well take advantage of the fact that your heels alternately peel off the ground as you walk — and use that for propulsion. (Could you walk very well if you didn't allow your heels to peel off and just slid your feet?)

Test this out with a grocery cart or even a lawn mower. (If you use a walker with wheels, you have immediate application.) Instead of having your arms do all the work:

- Allow your shoulders to relax.
- Stand close enough to the object you're pushing so that your elbows are bent about 90 degrees.
- Allow your hands and arms to simply be the connecting link between you and the cart.
- Allow your heels to alternately peel off the ground to propel you and the cart forward.

What about going upstairs or uphill? Let's experiment...

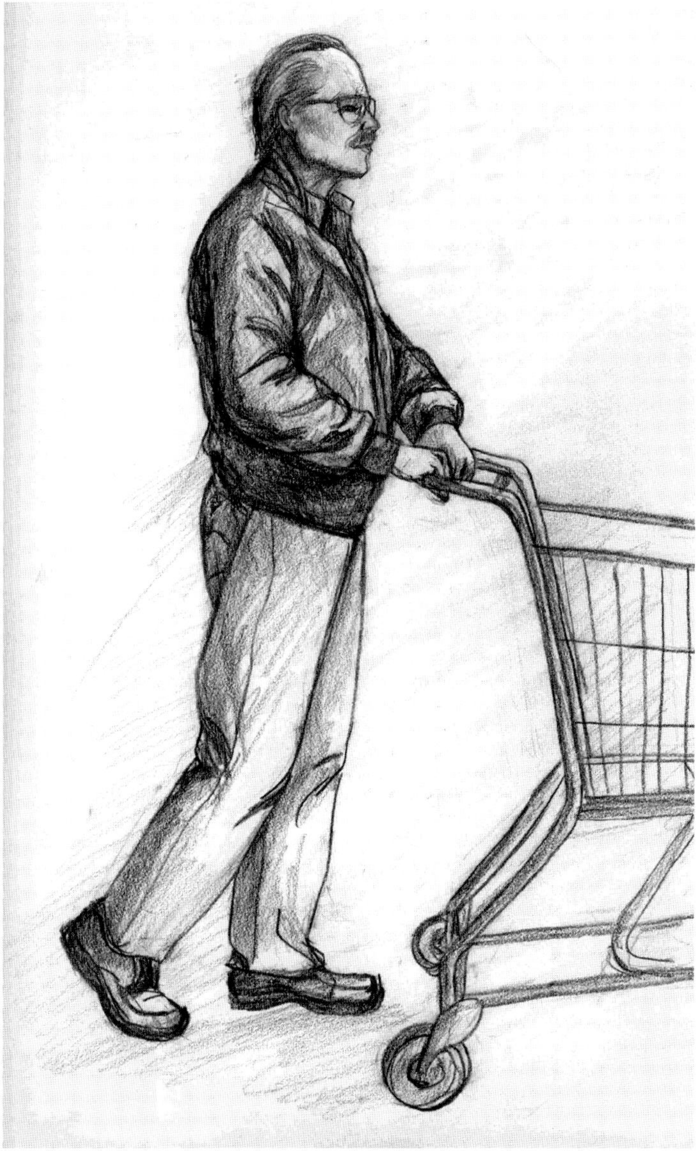

EXPERIMENT…

Can Your Foot that's Behind You Power You Up Stairs?

Equipment needed: bottom step of stairway or solidly-built step stool.

1. Stand facing bottom step of stairway (or step stool placed in front of countertop) with one hand resting on the banister (or both hands resting on the countertop).
2. Allow your shoulders and elbows to relax. For this experiment your arms and hands are to rest, not work.
3. With your arms remaining relaxed, have one foot pull you up on the stair or step stool, then return that foot to the floor. Do this several times with that same foot, noticing the amount of effort this takes.
4. Pause with both feet making solid contact with the floor.
5. With one hand resting on the banister (or both hands resting on

the countertop), your arms relaxed, start to lift that same foot while simultaneously allowing the heel of your other foot to peel off the floor; then let both feet rest solidly on the floor again. Do this several times and notice:

Does the lifting of the heel of the foot that remains on the floor help the other foot lift onto the stair?

6. To confirm for yourself what is most efficient, several times move up on to the stair or stepstool alternating between (a) having one foot pull you up and (b) having the other heel peel off the floor to propel you onto the stair or stepstool.

   Don't hold your breath through any of this so that you can determine which way of climbing allows you to breathe more easily.

   Notice which way is more comfortable for your back.

Throughout this book you'll discover that the dynamics that apply to walking down the sidewalk also apply to walking up stairs or uphill.

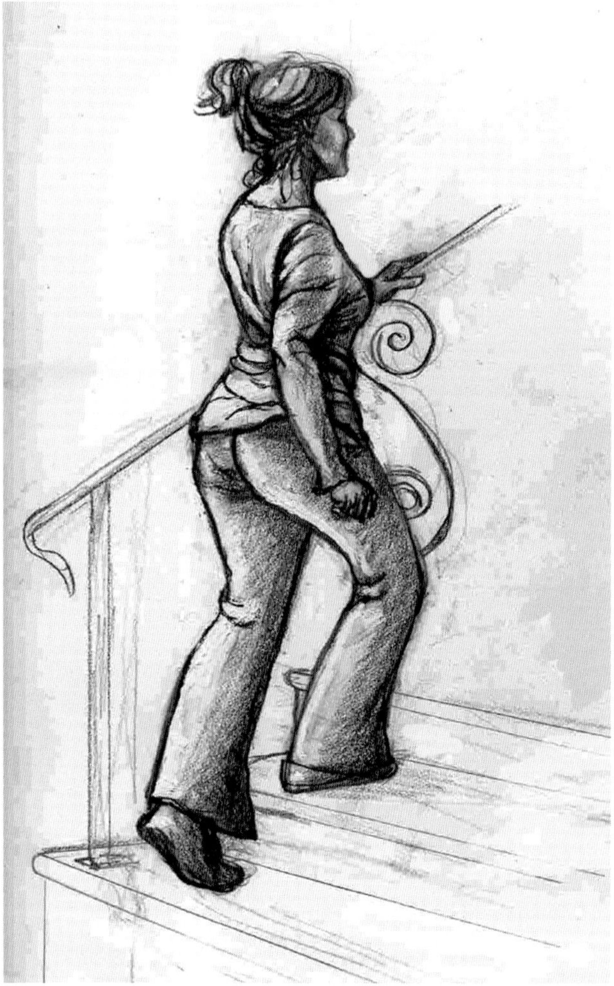

Whenever you walk uphill or climb stairs:

- Allow the heel of the foot that is behind you to peel off the ground to propel your body forward and to help your other foot move forward and up.
- Then allow the heel of the foot that just moved forward and up to peel off to continue propelling you forward.

The more you allow your feet and ankles to be flexible, the easier it is to take advantage of your heels leaving the ground to propel you forward — wherever you happen to be.

Propelling yourself forward — instead of drawing yourself forward — is powerful!

Third Step...
Fully Use Your Footprints

A healthy footprint indicates the path for healthful walking.

Only some of the bones in the foot participate in the footprint one sees when stepping out of water onto concrete. That footprint is the map for what we should be standing on when we come up from sitting to standing.

A healthy footprint is the imprint made by:

- calcaneus (heel),
- cuboid connecting calcaneus to 4th metatarsal
- length of 4th metatarsal
- head of 5th, 4th, 3rd, 2nd, and 1st metatarsals
- distal phalanges (beneath toenails)

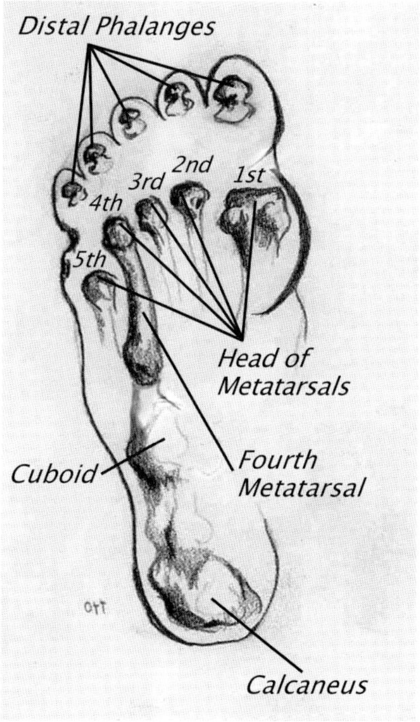

Bones involved in footprint, viewed from underneath

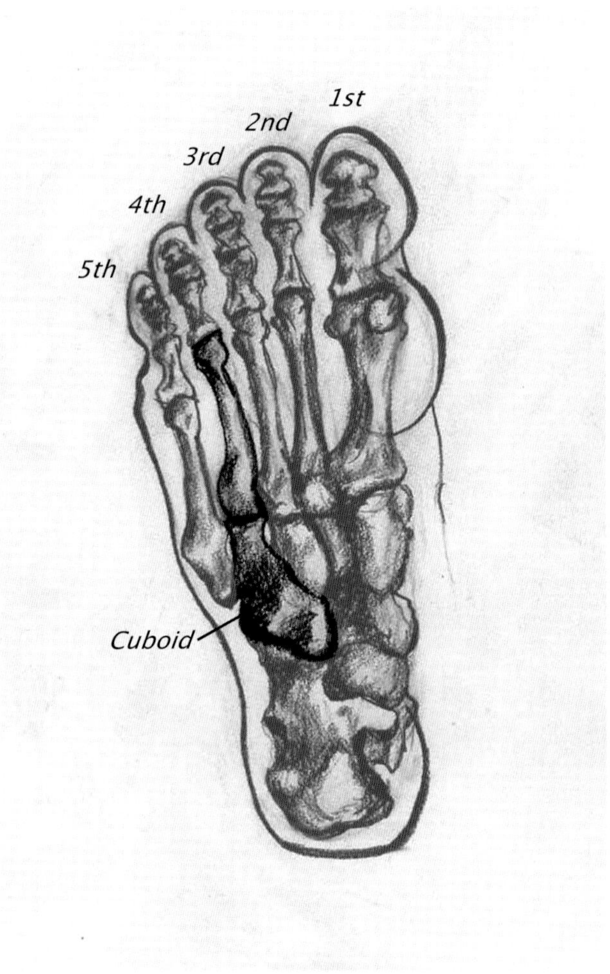

Bones of right foot viewed from underneath

Why the 4th metatarsal?

If you press too much into the 5th metatarsal, your foot will roll outward (supinated).

If the length of the 1st, 2nd, or even 3rd metatarsal is pressed into the ground, your foot will roll inward (pronated), decreasing the arches of your foot and increasing the chance of bunion formation.

While walking:

The gliding joints of the cuboid transmit the power from the heel peeling off the ground directly through the length of the 4th metatarsal.

The length of the 4th metatarsal levers you onto the "ball of your foot."

There's a split-second ripple effect from the head of the 4th metatarsal through the heads of the 3rd and 2nd — so that right at the power point when your heel peels off the ground to propel you forward, your middle three toes support your knee.

The job of your 1st and 5th toes is simply to be relaxed "outriggers" for balance. In fact, if you have the time to think about only one thing while walking — allow a space between your big toe and second toe on each foot *as each heel takes its turn to peel away from the ground*, and you will be following the path of your footprints.

Notice the spaces between the length of the bones of the toes. (What we call "toes" is less than one half the total length of our toes.) We weren't meant to wear shoes that squish those spaces!

If you don't allow healthful space between your big toe and second toe, and you don't allow the length of the 4th toe to lever you on to the metatarsal area — you may ("jaywalk") slide across your arch from the heel directly to the big toe, or worse, from the heel directly to the bunion.

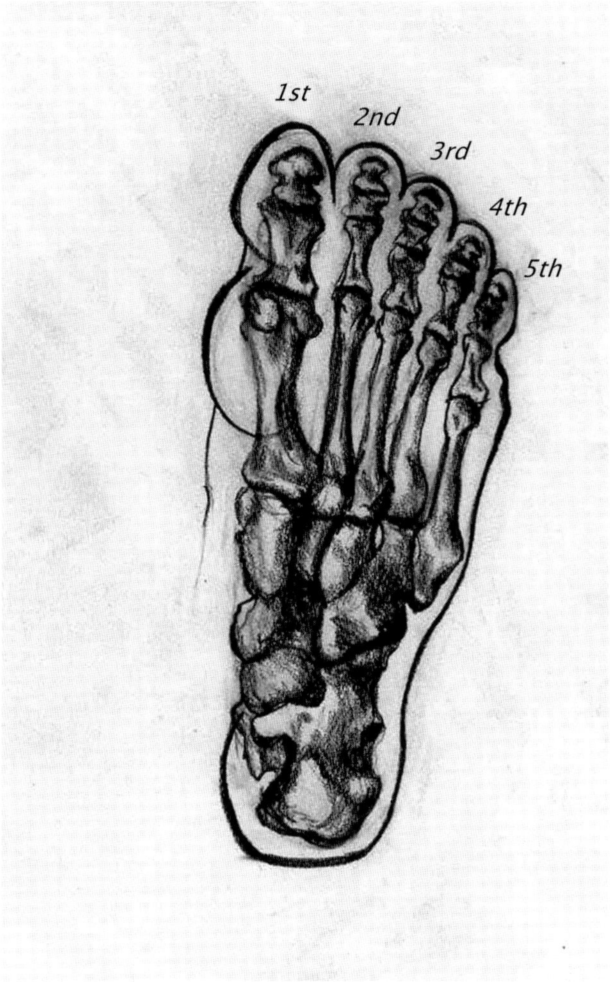

Bones of left foot viewed from underneath

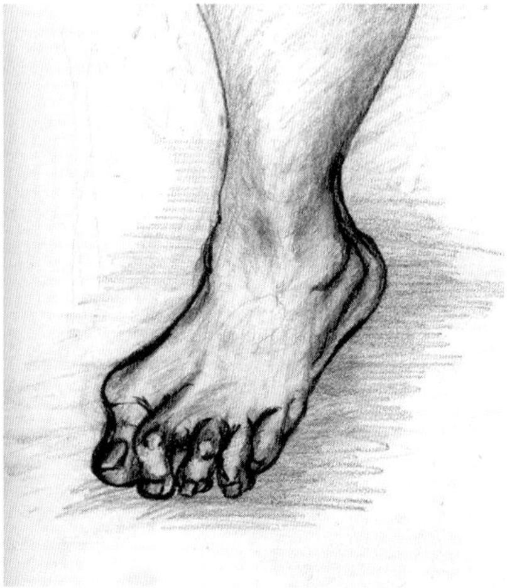

If you "jaywalk" across the arch of your foot:

- ⃠ You encourage bunions.

  A bunion is formed when the head of the first metatarsal is pushed sideways (medially) and the tip of the big toe moves toward the second toe. (If you push one end of a bone toward the midline of the body, the other end moves away from the center of the body.)

- ⃠ You diminish the medial (long) and transverse (crosswise) arches of your foot.

  The arches of your foot are not just there for aesthetics — they enable your walking to have springiness for comfort and power.

- ⃠ Your foot cannot fully support your knee.

In order to use your footprint fully, allow your feet and ankles the flexibility that nature intended.

The job description for your feet and ankles is to be as relaxed as possible. This is true whether you're walking across a street or traversing a mountain path.

It's not in your best interest to:

- ⃠ Curl your toes while you walk, which is like walking with your brakes on.
- ⃠ Pull up your toes as you walk, which also slows you down and exerts unnecessary pressure on the heads of your metatarsals — sometimes causing "the ball" of the foot to be very tender, or
- ⃠ Stiffen through your ankles, which also interferes with comfortable, efficient walking.

In fact, flexibility through your feet and ankles is so important that a "drop foot" (flexion is impossible or nearly impossible) is problematic to walking only when you step far ahead of yourself.

Flexibility through your feet and ankles also allows you to walk up and down stairs more smoothly, more easily. If you wish to, experiment to see if this is true for you:

EXPERIMENT...

Can Allowing Your Ankles To Relax Make Walking Up Stairs Easier?

1. Pour water into a cup, about halfway, i.e. not close to the top of the cup.
2. Stand near the bottom step with one hand holding the handrail, the other hand holding the cup.
3. Stand still until the water basically stops moving.
4. Stiffen your ankles and feet. Then holding onto the bannister, walk up a few stairs with your feet and ankles held stiffly.

   Notice the degree to which the water sloshes side-to-side inside the cup.

5. Again stand near the bottom step with one hand holding the handrail, the other hand holding the cup, waiting until the water basically stops moving.
6. With your feet and ankles as relaxed and flexible as possible, walk up a few stairs while holding on to the banister and watching the water in the cup.

   Notice the degree to which the water moves side-to-side inside the cup now.

Do you think walking — whether across the room or up a mountain trail — might be more gentle on your body if you allow your feet and ankles to be relaxed?

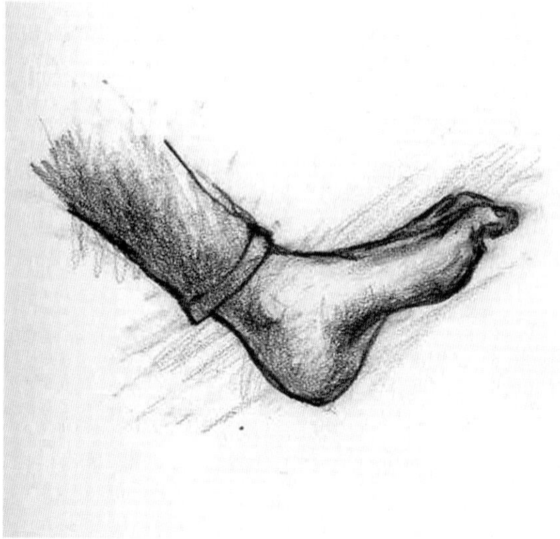

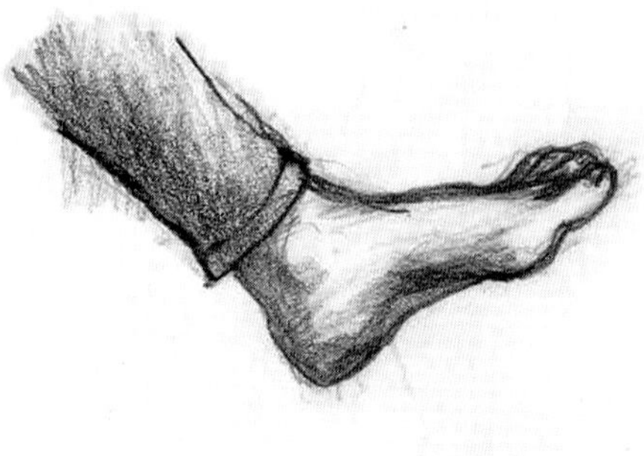

Exercise Three... Flexibility through your Toes

1. While lying in bed or sitting in a chair with your shoes removed, pretend to pick up a marble with your toes.

   Allow your ankle to bend (dorsi-flex) as your toes curl to "pick up the marble."

   Could you do this if you didn't allow the "ball of your foot" to participate?

   Since the goal here is to enhance flexibility — not to encourage tightening — go into this curling slowly and luxuriously (like an animal arching its back to stretch upon awakening).
2. Allow your toes to relax into lengthening after each time you curl your toes.
3. Alternate between "picking up the marble" and relaxing your toes.
4. Spend twice as much time relaxing your toes — i.e. if you take three counts to "pick up the marble," take six counts to relax.

Exercise Four… Foot and Ankle Flexibility

1. Stand with your feet parallel to each other, not quite as far apart as the distance between your shoulders.
2. Peel one heel off the ground and then allow it to return to the ground. The front third of the bottom of that foot ("ball" of the foot and "toes") remains on the ground.
3. Slowly alternate peeling one heel, then the other, off the ground. Wait until the first heel returns to the ground before you lift the other heel.

   Each time one of your heels peels off the ground, allow that knee to move forward. (If you don't allow the knee to bend as the heel below it peels off the ground, you'll end up "standing on your toes" instead of relaxing through your toes.)

   When one of your heels peels off the ground, allow the front of that ankle to lengthen.

   Allow the length of the 4th metatarsal to lever you onto the "ball" (heads of your metatarsals).

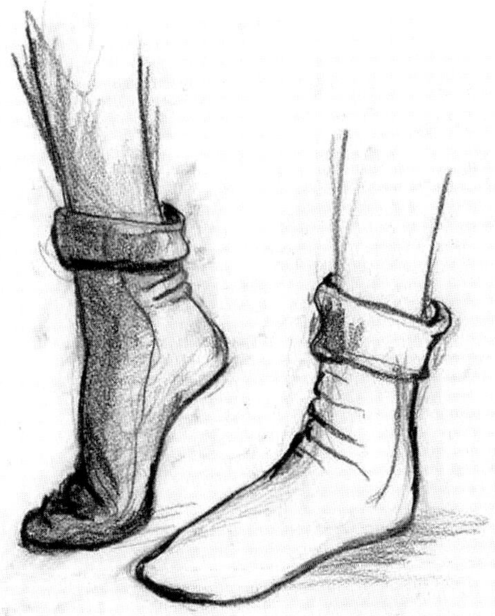

Each time one of your heels peels off the ground, allow a space between your "big toe" and 2nd toe and between your "little toe" and 4th toe — to allow your middle three toes to support your knee.

Allowing your 1st (big) toe and 5th (little) toe to allow your middle three toes to support your knee, means allowing relaxed lengthening through *all* of your toes.

The human foot is designed for relaxed lengthening through the toes and for bend-ability where the heads of the metatarsals meet the phalanges. Both of these enable your heels to peel off the ground for comfortable, powerful walking.

Make sure every pair of shoes you own has enough:

- toe-room to allow your toes to spread into relaxed lengthening, and
- bend-ability to allow you to move onto the ball of your foot every time your heel peels off the ground behind you.

If you want to walk faster — instead of making your legs work harder, allow your feet and ankles to be more flexible.

FOURTH STEP...
Allow Your Knees to be Supported by Your Feet

While walking, knee and foot alignment is extremely important for the health of your back and hip joints, as well as for the comfort and safety of your knees.

You're already taking steps to protect your knees if you're following through with the FIRST, SECOND, and THIRD STEPS in this book.

In FIRST STEP you learned it's important to allow the front of you to lengthen instead of crunch. Look again at Moshe Feldenkrais's "pretend to jump" trick (pages 10-12), the result of which provides maximum safety for your knees.

In SECOND STEP you learned that the most efficient way to walk is to allow your stride to be under and behind you, instead of striding out ahead of yourself.

When you stride out ahead of yourself (the way many of us thought we were supposed to walk) there is a moment when you have to pull your body weight over your heel and onto that front foot. That moment is vulnerable for the knee of your leg that is out in front.

However, when your stride is behind you, as each foot takes its turn to land directly underneath you it instantaneously supports that knee.

And, even though the foot that is behind you is in the process of powering you forward as your heel peels off the ground, that back knee can fully be supported by your middle three toes.

When your stride is behind you, the front leg (directly underneath you) is safely supporting most of your weight.

THIRD STEP taught you awareness of fully using your footprints. Your knee will not be supported if you "jaywalk" across your foot instead of following your footprint (page 26). However, if you allow the length of your 4th toe to lever you onto the "ball" of your foot as your heel leaves the ground, your knee will be perfectly supported (page 24).

When your stride is behind you and you allow the length of your 4th toe to lever you onto the "ball" of the foot as each foot takes its turn behind you:

- your knee and foot will be perfectly aligned in that moment when each foot is behind you propelling you forward
- your knee and foot will also be effortlessly and perfectly aligned when they take their turn to be directly underneath you supporting the weight of your body.

Putting your stride behind you allows your knees to be securely supported by your feet, every step of the way.

Dr. Feldenkrais applied engineering principles to his own body in every moment, in every movement.

Dr. Moshe Feldenkrais, the originator of the Feldenkrais Method® of Somatic Education upon which this book is based, had extremely damaged knees from a soccer accident that happened in his early twenties. However, in his late seventies, while engrossed in conversation, he could stand up from sitting in an overstuffed chair *smoothly and comfortably — ready to walk* — in spite of being overweight and having a history of severe pain.

Would you like to learn one of Moshe's "engineering" tricks to help your knee alignment? This trick is based on the idea of a circus acrobat balancing in a handstand on another performer's knees. Feldenkrais used that image to organize himself so that his feet optimally supported his knees while sitting and before standing up.

EXPERIMENT:
Are Your Feet Supporting Your Knees?

1. As you're sitting, notice if an imaginary acrobat could safely maintain a hand-stand on your knees.

   The answer is no if you're not allowing the footprint (page 23) of your right foot and your left foot to sink into the ground.

The answer is no if your knees are in closer than your feet or out farther than your feet.

2. Lift one knee a little bit and then let it drop so that foot sinks to make solid contact with the ground. Then, do the same with the other leg and foot.

   Can you sense that when each footprint is solidly on the ground, your legs are organized so that an *imaginary* acrobat could balance in a handstand on your knees?

   Notice that you don't have to tense your feet or leg muscles to maintain this organization.

3. A few times alternate between this way of sitting with your feet solid on the ground and your habitual way of sitting.

   In which position are you more ready to move up to standing?

4. Alternate standing up from your habitual way of sitting and standing up from sitting organized as if someone could do a handstand on your knees.

   Notice which way allows you to stand up with the least amount of effort.

   Notice which way allows you to stand up the most comfortably.

Exercise Five... Your Footprints Can Support Your Knees While Walking

1. Remove your shoes so that you can experience this lesson stocking-footed or barefooted.
2. Sit on a firm chair with your feet flat on the floor and parallel to each other about your shoulders' distance apart. (If you need to, place a book under each foot so that each foot has a solid surface.)
3. Notice what parts of your right foot and your left foot are actually making contact with that solid surface. Don't change anything right away, just notice:

   Are your two footprints mirrors of each other?

   If not, what's different about the way each foot makes contact with the "ground." ("Ground" here refers to the surface your foot is resting on, even if it's a book.)

4. Without shifting yourself in any way, notice if one knee angles outward or inward more than the other.
5. Roll on the bottom of your feet just a small amount outward so that you're a bit more on the outside edge; then roll your feet back to their starting position. Do this slowly several times.

   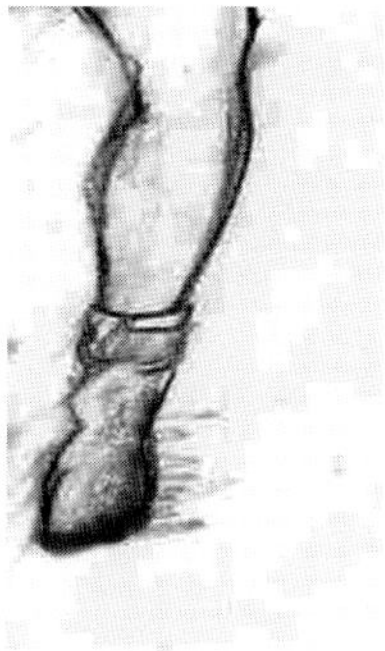

   Notice what happens to the position of your knees each time your feet roll outward.

   Imagine what would happen to your knee if you stood up with one foot rolled even a little bit outward.

   Imagine what would happen through your knee if you walked up stairs or up a hill or ramp with that foot rolled even a little bit outward.

   Imagine what would happen to your knee if you walked down the sidewalk with this foot even a little bit rolled outward.
6. Roll on the bottom of your feet just a small amount inward so that you're a bit more on the inside edge of your feet; then roll your feet back

to their starting position. Do this slowly several times.

Notice what happens to the position of your knees each time your feet roll inward.

Imagine what would happen to your knees if you stood up with your feet rolled even a little bit inward.

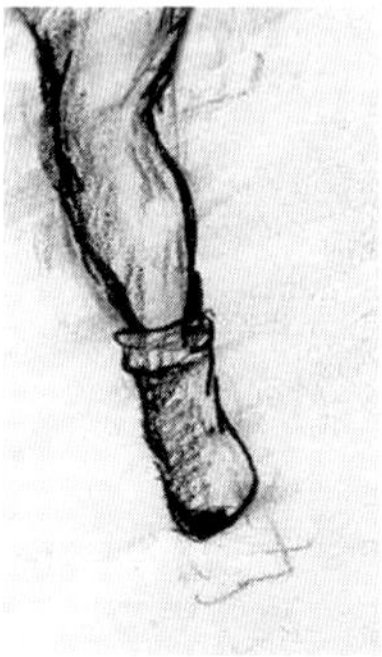

Imagine what would happen to your knees if you walked up stairs or up a hill or ramp with one or both feet rolled even a little bit inward.

Imagine what would happen to your knees if you walked down the sidewalk with one or both feet rolled even a little bit inward.

7. Now allow each foot's ideal footprint (page 23) to make contact with "the ground" — i.e. the heel, length of 4th metatarsal, "ball of the foot" area, and the pads directly underneath each toenail.

   Notice the position of your knees.

   Can you imagine that your knees would be safer if you stood up on each ideal footprint instead of rolling outward or inward on your footprints?

8. With one foot, lift your heel, which lifts the heel-end of the length of your 4th (next to "little") toe, to lever you onto the "ball of your foot" (actually the heads of all five metatarsals). Then allow that heel to return to "the ground."

   Do this several times sensing how your knee is supported through the whole process.

9. Continue with #8, alternating between squeezing your toes as your heel lifts and then allowing your toes to relax and spread as your heel lifts.

   Notice if your lower leg muscles don't have to tense as much when you lift your heel with your toes relaxed away from each other.

   Notice if your middle three toes, from the ball of your foot to the bottom of the ends of your toes, can solidly and effortlessly support your knee when your toes are relaxed away from each other.

Does this help you understand why you don't want your shoes or stockings to squeeze your toes together?

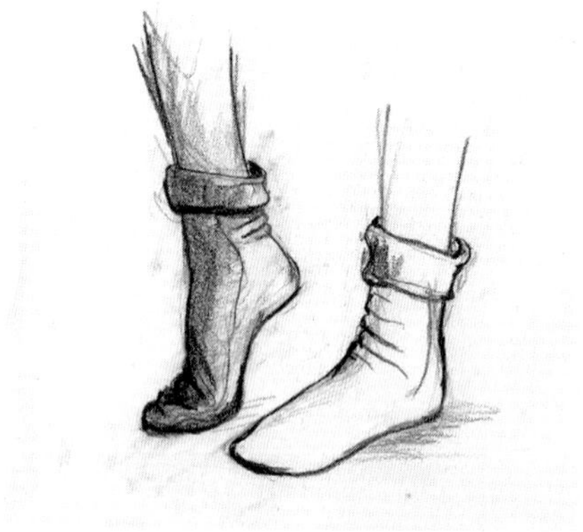

10. With your toes relaxed, lift your heel allowing the length of your 4th metatarsal to lever you onto the heads of your middle three metatarsals consecutively — so that your 4th toe, then, less than a split second later, your 3rd and your 2nd toes (all three middle) support your knee.

11. With your other foot, follow this ideal path of your footprint as your heel leaves the ground. Do this several times until the path for this foot is clear.

12. Alternate having the heel of one foot peel off the ground and then the other heel, making sure that you follow the above instructions in #10 for each foot so that each knee is fully supported.

13. Now stand up and slowly, in place, alternate having one heel and then the other heel peel off the ground, adding awareness of the length of the 4th metatarsal levering you onto the "ball" of your foot, so that right before each heel returns to the ground, your middle three toes are fully supporting that knee.

    Be sure that you allow your toes to be relaxed.

14. Walk across the room allowing a space between your big toe & 2nd toe and between your 5th & 4th toes when

each foot takes its turn behind you, as each heel takes its turn to peel away from the ground.

Sense how both knees are supported through every step when you follow each footprint as each heel takes its turn to peel away from the ground.

Instead of trying to control a wayward habitually turned-out leg and foot by strengthening your adductor muscles or trying to correct a habitually turned-in leg and foot with your abductor muscles, you can simply follow the logic of your skeletal footprints.

When you follow your skeletal "blueprint," your muscles will participate as Nature intended.

When your skeleton is well organized, your muscles don't have to exert as much effort to help you move powerfully.

"Skeletal engineering" can also be applied to walking downhill and down stairs:

If your back, hips, or knees are bothering you, it's possible (safer and often more comfortable) to walk down stairs backward. (You can see the step below you through the window formed by the arm of your hand on the banister.)

Walking down stairs backward encourages your pelvis to reposition so that your coccyx (tail bone) is released — resulting in a more relaxed spine and more comfortable bend-ability through your hip joints and knees.

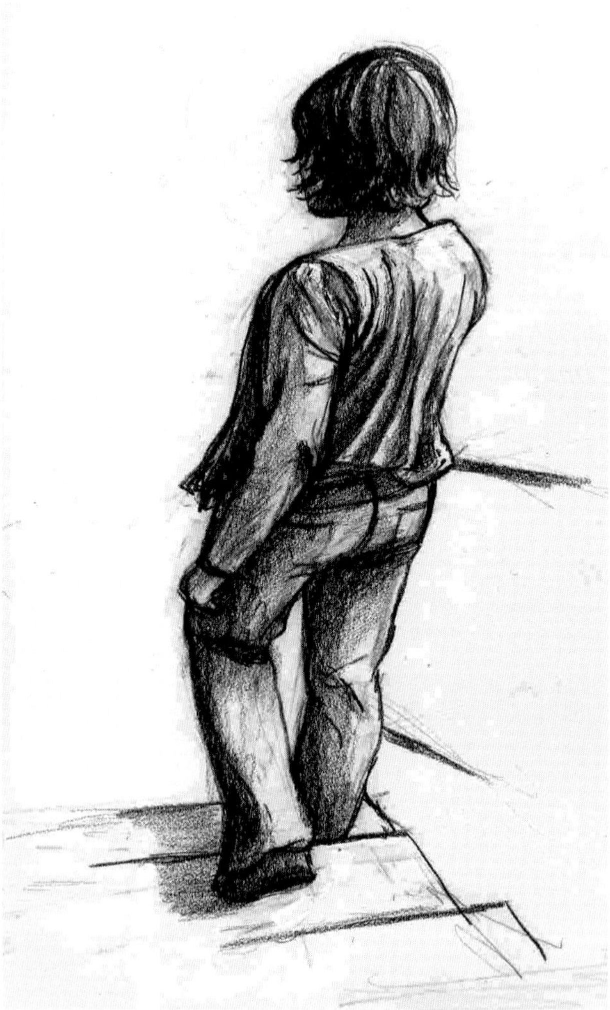

Walking down stairs facing forward, there is a moment when your back leg is supporting your weight in a bent-knee position. You want to move out of that as quickly as possible!

- For the sake of your knees, it's imperative that you allow your toes and your ankles to be as relaxed as possible so that your heel can immediately peel off the stair behind you.
- It's also in your best interest to allow space between your 1st & 2nd toes and the 5th & 4th toes as your heel is peeling off the stair behind you — so that your middle three toes can fully support your knee through that vulnerable bent-knee moment while walking down stairs.

"Skeletal engineering" can be applied to every aspect of your life.

FIFTH STEP…

Allow your Pelvis to Help you Walk

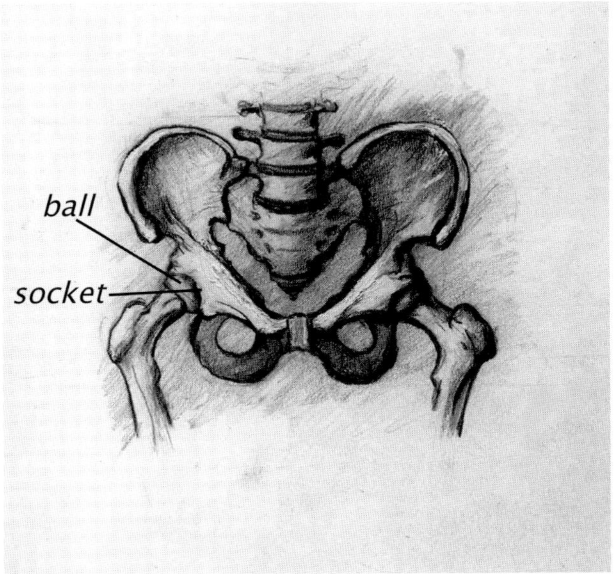

Your pelvis is a bony bowl that includes the right and left sockets of your right and left hip ball-and-socket joints. The "ball" is the uppermost and innermost part of your thigh bone (femur).

The following is very important information for everyone — especially for those who have arthritis in a hip joint or have had a hip replacement: Your hip joints actually receive less wear and tear when you allow your pelvis to rotate subtly as you walk.

As you're walking, the socket of your ball-and-socket hip joint needs to travel with the ball. If you don't allow that to happen, your hip joints are more — not less — vulnerable.

Do you think it might be easier to have a generous stride if you allow your pelvis to rotate? Remember, stride is simply the forward/backward distance between your feet as you're walking.

EXPERIMENT...

Can Your Pelvis Help Your Stride Be Behind You?

1. Stand facing a countertop with both hands resting on the countertop, close enough to the countertop that your elbows are slightly bent when you're upright (i.e. not slouching or bending forward).
2. Place your feet parallel to each other, as if on narrow parallel tracks.
3. While remaining upright (not bending forward) slide your left foot backward on its "track" a few times noticing how far backward that foot can *comfortably* travel.
4. Again, slide your left foot backward on its "track," this time allowing your pelvis to simultaneously rotate a bit to the left so that your left hip joint is also traveling backward.

5. Alternate sliding your left foot backward with your pelvis rotating and without your pelvis rotating.

   Which way allows your foot to travel back farther and more easily?

If you have lots of energy but often find it challenging to cross the street before the "Walk" sign changes to "Don't Walk," you probably are not allowing your pelvis to rotate as you walk.

It's important to allow the rotation of your pelvis to travel up your spine into your upper back instead of getting stuck in your lower back.

If you try to make your pelvis rotate in isolation, the twist happens in your lumbar spine; instead, ***allow the rotation to flow up into your rib basket!***

Your rib "cage" really is a rib "basket," constructed strong enough to protect its contents (heart and lungs) yet pliable enough to allow quite a bit of flexibility. Your ribs are *jointed* to your spinal vertebrae in the back of your rib basket, and connected to your sternum (breastbone) in front with a *generous* amount of pliable cartilage.

Because of its unique construction, your thorax (rib basket) can readily twist into asymmetry then settle back into symmetry when you stop twisting.

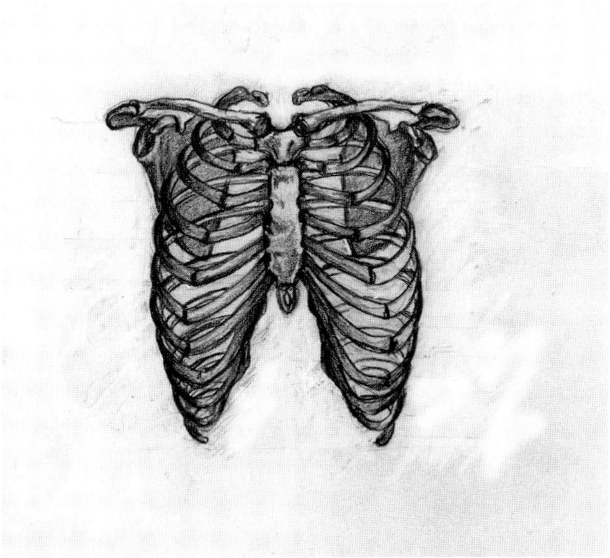

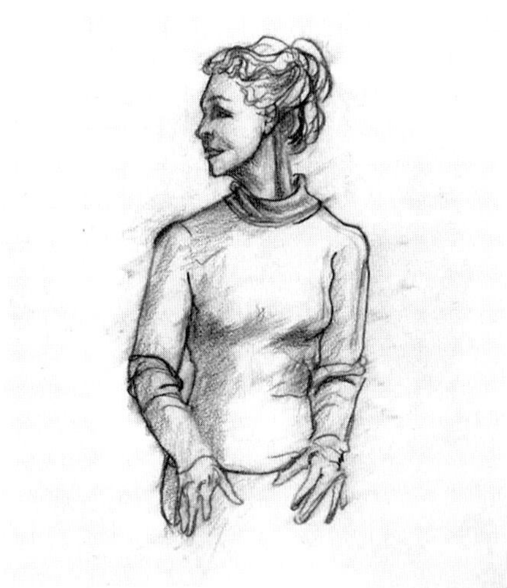

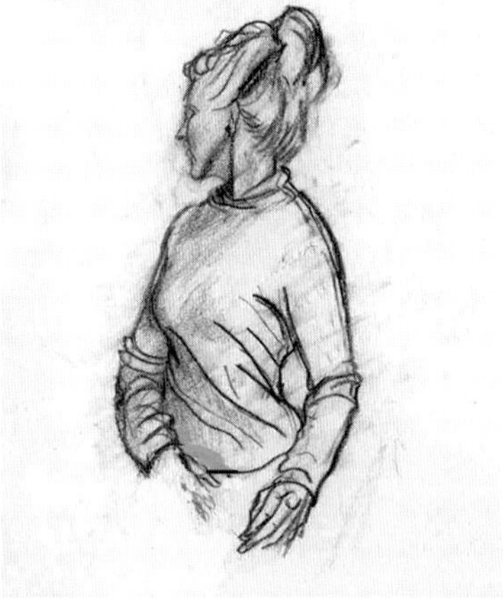

Do you think having a pliable rib basket might help you determine whether it's safe to cross a busy street?

To test this out:

Look over your shoulder pretending your thorax is a rib "cage."

Then, wiggle out and look over your shoulder again knowing that your thorax is a pliable rib basket.

For flexible movement through your rib basket, take a moment to discover your rib wiggle potential:

- Pretend that you're drying your upper back by moving your upper back side-to-side instead of moving the towel.
- Pretend that you're a bear scratching its upper back against a tree.
- Pretend that you're flossing your ribs.

Because your ribs are connected to twelve of your spinal vertebrae, every time you wiggle your ribs you ceate gentle movement along the entire length of your spine.

EXPERIMENT...

Can Your Rib "Basket" Help Your Pelvis Lengthen Your Stride Behind You?

1. Again, stand facing a countertop with both hands resting on the countertop, close enough to the countertop that your elbows are slightly bent when you're upright (i.e. not slouching or bending forward).
2. Place your feet parallel to each other, as if on narrow parallel tracks.
3. While remaining upright (not bending forward) slide one foot backward on its "track," allowing your pelvis to rotate so the hip joint on that same side also travels back.
4. Slide that foot forward until it is once again under you, then slide your other foot back on its "parallel track." Alternate this way.

   Each time your left foot slides backward and your pelvis rotates a bit to the left, allow the rotation to travel up your spine through your rib basket so that your ribs rotate a bit under your arms.

Allow your rib basket asymmetry to allow your spine to respond to this rotation of your pelvis all the way up between your shoulder blades.

Each time your right foot slides backward and your pelvis rotates a bit to the right, allow the rotation to travel up your spine through your rib basket so that your ribs rotate a bit under your arms.

5. Briefly, for the purposes of this experiment, pretend your rib basket is an immovable rib "cage" as your feet take turns sliding back on the "parallel tracks."

   Notice if there's a sizable difference in how far backward your feet can travel when you restrict the potential of your rib basket to help your pelvis and spine rotate.

   Wiggle out so that your rib basket can once again can have its full potential of pliability.

6. Allow your pelvis and your rib basket to rotate as you resume gently sliding one foot and then the other backward.

7. A few times, alternate between #5 and #6 to verify for yourself which way is more effective and which way is more comfortable.

Exercise Seven... Freeing Up Your Built-In Flexibility for Healthful Walking

1. Lie on your back on your bed, with your knees bent and supported by your feet.
2. In your "mind's eye" sense the entire length of your spine, from your coccyx/tailbone to the top of your neck up under your skull.
3. Without sliding or lifting your feet, roll the bowl of your pelvis a little bit to the right and left.

   Notice that your legs also move since your legs are connected to your pelvis through your ball-and-socket hip joints.
4. As you continue gently rolling your pelvis a bit left and right, notice that your lumbar (lower back) vertebrae want to follow the rolling of your sacrum (five spinal vertebrae fused to each other in the center back of your pelvis).

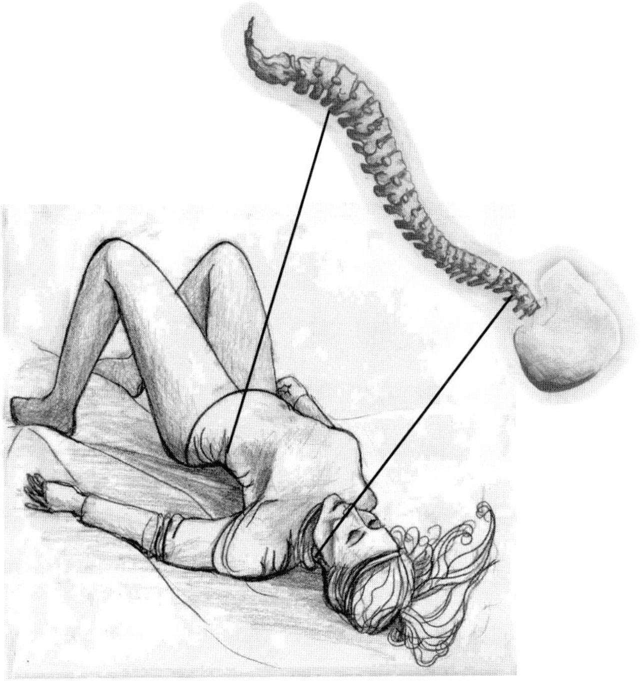

Your lumbar (lower back) vertebrae have to follow, as your spine is a continuum from your coccyx (tailbone) to the top of your neck.

Even though sections of the spine are frequently labeled separately for reference and clarity, your spine is a continuum.

5. Pause, and remember that you want your pelvis to rotate while walking, but don't want the twist to happen directly in your lumbar vertebrae. Instead, the twist can happen above — in your thoracic (rib) vertebrae.
6. With your fingertips, trace the length of your sternum (breastbone).

   Directly below your throat is a bony notch, the middle of which is the top of your sternum.

   Your lower ribs merge up to the bottom of your sternum.

   The length of your sternum is about the distance between your thumb and fifth finger when they are stretched away from each other.

Since your ribs connect your sternum ("breastbone") to your spine, you can use your sternum as a landmark for what's happening through your thoracic (rib) vertebrae.

7. Resume gently rolling your sacrum left and right — allowing the bottom of your sternum to follow.
8. Allow your neck and shoulders to relax so that the gentle rotational movement of your pelvis travels up your spine between your scapulae (shoulder blades).

In order for the bottom of your sternum to follow your pelvis, your whole rib basket needs to be freely pliable to allow asymmetry.

Exercise Eight... "Walking" while Lying on a Blanket Roller

Equipment needed: one twin-size blanket, thick but soft textured is ideal.

1. Fold a twin-sized blanket width-wise and then length-wise so it's a quarter of its original size. Roll it from the longer side like a jelly-roll cake.
2. Place the rolled blanket on the middle of your bed so that you can lie on your side with the back of your head and your entire spine down to your coccyx (tailbone) touching the blanket roller.
3. With your knees bent, roll up onto the rolled blanket so that this blanket roller can support you from the top of your head to your coccyx.
4. Position your feet on the bed wider than the blanket roller so that your feet can solidly support your bent knees. Allow your arms to relax to either side of you on the bed.

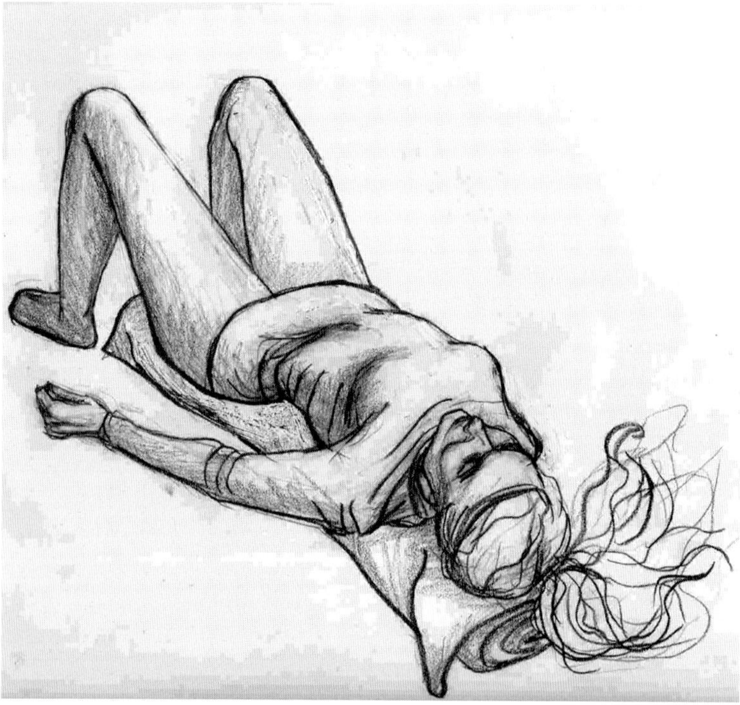

The more you allow yourself to relax, the more benefit you'll receive from this exercise.

5. Take a moment to sense how your sacrum (base of your spine in the center back of your pelvis), your whole spine, and the back of your head can be supported by the blanket roller.

   Allow yourself to be so relaxed that your rib basket molds around the blanket roller and your shoulders drape over the blanket roller.

6. Allow one side of your pelvis to give in to gravity, sinking a bit toward the bed.

   Notice that as one side sinks, the other side rises — because your pelvis is essentially a bowl.

7. Now allow the raised side of your pelvis to give in to gravity, noticing that as this side sinks the other side passively rises.

8. Gently let your pelvis alternate this way ("seesawing") — one side passively being lifted as the other side sinks.

9. Rest for a moment, your feet positioned to support your bent knees so solidly that you don't have to tense through your legs and hip joints.

10. Resume the "seesaw" motion, noticing what happens with your knees as your pelvis sinks a little bit to one side and then to the other.

    Do your knees move side-to-side as your pelvis seesaws?

    Discover if you can minimize the side-to-side knee movement — not by tightening muscles, but with "skeletal-engineering" placement of your feet to support the bridges of your knees.

You'll momentarily discover that instead of the knees simply falling side-to-side, the movement can evolve to simulate "walking."

11. Since the pliability of your rib basket and flexibility of your spine are important elements in your pelvis helping your legs walk, wiggle side-to-side through your rib basket while on the blanket roller.

    Allow this rib wiggle to travel the whole length of your spine, down to the bottom of your coccyx and up under your skull, so that your pelvis and your skull respond.

12. As you resume the seesaw motion of your pelvis, allow the bottom of your sternum (breastbone) to be passively drawn to follow the side-to-side sinking of your pelvis.

Simply allow one side and then the other side to use gravity to sink. (None of this is intentional lifting.).

As the left side of your pelvis sinks, allow the bottom of your sternum to be passively drawn to the left.

As the right side of your pelvis sinks, allow the bottom of your sternum to be passively drawn to the right.

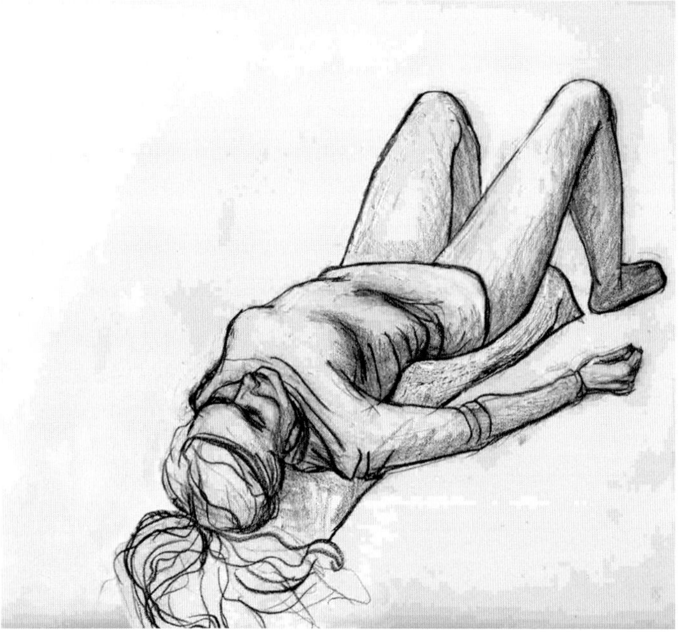

13. Using good skeletal engineering in your foot and knee placement so that your hip joints can remain relaxed, continue the "seesaw" motion of your pelvis while paying particular attention to your right hip joint.

    Each time the left side of your pelvis sinks, the right side of your pelvis passively rises so your right hip joint is passively raised.

    Each time your right hip joint is passively raised — if your right knee doesn't fall to the left — your right knee "lengthens" forward toward your toes. (Your feet stay in place the whole time.)

14. Shift your attention to your left hip joint as your pelvis seesaws.

    Each time the left side of your pelvis passively rises as the right side of your pelvis sinks, your left hip joint is passively raised and — if your left knee doesn't fall to the right —

your left knee “lengthens” (”walks”) forward toward your toes.

Your feet stay in place so that your knees are fully supported throughout.

15. As a brief experiment, don’t let your sternum (breastbone) move as you seesaw your pelvis.

    Can your pelvis alternately “walk” your knees very well (if at all) when you don’t allow mobility through your rib basket?

Can you now understand, even more fully, why we need to allow the front of us to be lengthened and relaxed instead of contracted while walking?

16. Resume allowing your rib basket to freely allow the bottom of your sternum to follow the rolling of your pelvis so that you can effortlessly “walk” your knees.

17. As you allow the seesaw motion of your pelvis to alternately “walk” each knee, in your “mind’s-eye” imagination translate this movement that’s happening while you’re lying horizontal on the blanket roller into upright walking.

    You are now “walking” with your stride behind you. The hip that is sinking (moving backward) is lifting (moving forward) the other hip which “walks” its knee forward.

Once again, your rib basket is allowing the movement in your sacrum to travel up your spine to between your scapulae so that your thoracic vertebrae can help your lumbar vertebrae safely (and passively) follow the roll of your pelvis.

18. When you're ready, slowly roll off the blanket roller.
19. Remain as relaxed as possible as you come up to standing. Then notice your posture.

    Sense the length of you now — through both the front of your body and the back of your body.
20. Without tensing muscles, allow your torso to be relaxed and tall so that your pelvis can freely rotate to walk you across the room or down a hallway.

Most powerful animals moving through their territory allow the pelvis to move.

If the seam of your slacks that is directly over your sacrum is just staying still while you walk, your pelvis is not rotating to help walk your legs — making your hip joints and knees more vulnerable.

You want to allow that seam and your sacrum to rotate a bit back to the left and alternately back to the right, to help one foot and then the other travel behind you, to power you forward!

Comfortable, powerful, even graceful, movement is directly related to relaxed mobility of the pelvis.

SIXTH STEP...

Allow your Upper Body to Help you Walk

Yes, your upper body can help your walking be more balanced and efficient. It's not just your arm swing that helps power you forward — it's your scapulae (shoulder blades) sliding over your rib basket!

In order for your scapulae to slide, your clavicles (collarbones) and the top of your sternum (breastbone) also need to be free to move, so you definitely need a pliable rib basket.

Allowing yourself to lengthen in relaxed upright posture (from the bottom up pages 3–5) enables all of this to happen.

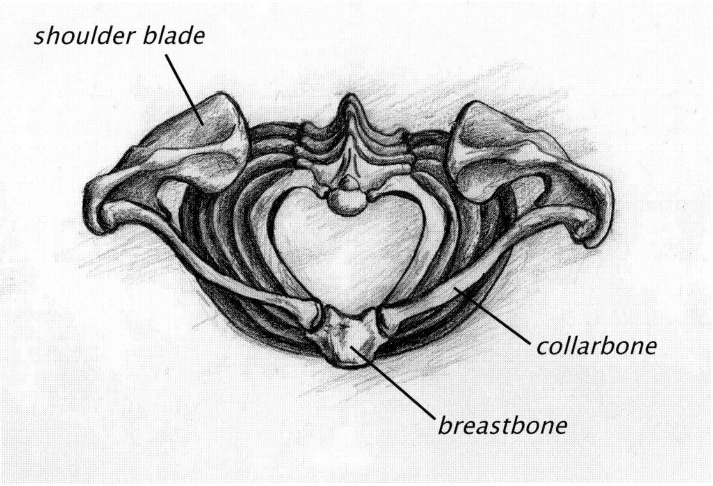

EXPERIMENT…
Can Your Upper Body Really Power Your Legs?

1. Stand next to a countertop, your body positioned sideways to the countertop so that the leg with which you're going to kick is away from the countertop. Let your hand that is closest to the countertop rest on that surface.
2. Without allowing your upper body or arms to move, kick an imaginary ball.

   How much power can you muster when you don't allow your upper body to participate?
3. This time as you kick the imaginary ball, continue to not allow any movement in your upper body — simply pull your arm (on the same side of your body as your kicking leg) back as that leg kicks forward.

   How much power does your kick have if you only move the arm, not the shoulder?

4. Now, as you kick forward with that same leg, allow your scapula ("shoulder blade" on the same side of your body as your kicking leg) to simultaneously slide over the back of your rib basket toward your spine — taking the elbow on the same side of your body backward as your leg kicks forward.

   How powerful was your kick this time?

5. Alternate between #2, #3, and #4 to confirm for yourself which way gives you the most powerful kick.

Soccer players moving the ball down the field, and the place kicker who powerfully kicks a football through the goal posts for the extra point, wouldn't be playing on the professional level if they kicked while keeping the upper body still.

This absolutely applies to walking. First of all, if you use your shoulders too powerfully, you'll end up kicking your legs out ahead.

Since you now know it's in your best interest to have your stride under and behind you instead of kicking out ahead — let your shoulders relax.

If you muscularly hold your scapulae to your rib basket as if they were one unit, yet use your shoulders powerfully while walking, your torso will follow your shoulders — i.e. as your right shoulder moves backward, the right side of your pelvis will also move backward (at the exact moment you need the right side of your pelvis to move forward to take your right leg forward to be directly under you).

The key is to allow your scapulae to slide over your rib basket.

Many of us as children were taught to keep our scapulae "glued" to our backs for "good" posture. "Don't let your little wings stick out." That "glue" (muscular tension) often remains into adulthood.

Your shoulders don't have to work hard to help you walk.

Let's take a moment to be even more clear about how you're skeletally connected.

Your scapula cannot slide unless your clavicle ("collarbone") goes along. This means that the front of your shoulder needs to be relaxed and open (not crunched) in order for your scapula to slide back.

Since the inner end of each clavicle is connected to your sternum, a sunken chest can trap your clavicles, which in turn inhibits the movement of your scapulae. (Yet another good reason for allowing the front of you to be lengthened, not crunched, as you walk.)

Looking at this illustration of a front view of the rib basket, can you understand why the following exercise to free up your sternum, clavicles, and scapulae, and spine is named "The Butterfly"?

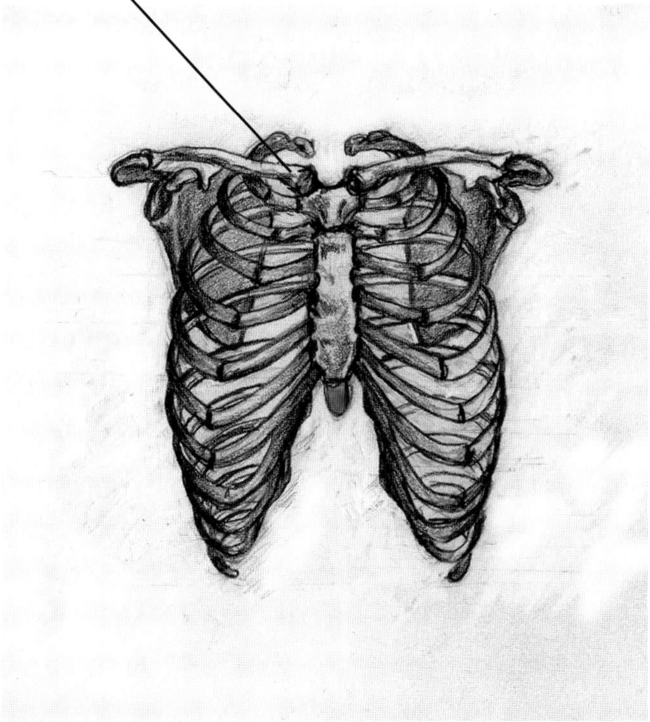

Exercise Nine... The Butterfly

1. Sit on a firm chair with your feet flat on the floor, placed a comfortable distance apart, parallel to each other.
2. Collapse your chest so that your sternum (the butterfly's body) sinks into you.

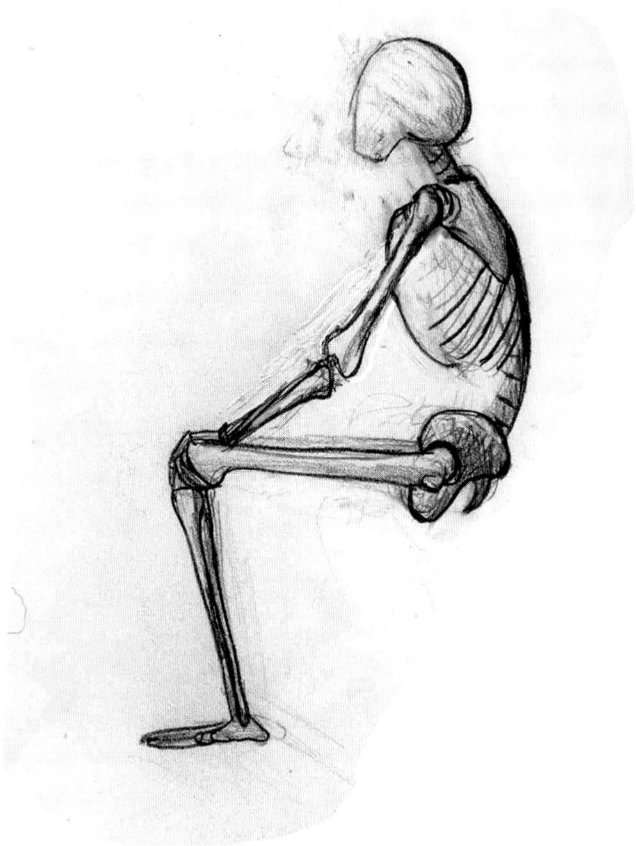

This moves your sternum backward a bit toward your spine, causing your corresponding section of spine between your scapulae to move backward.

This backward movement also causes your ribs (the butterfly's wings), which are attached to your sternum with flexible cartilage, to fold forward a bit.

The inner ends of your clavicles (the butterfly's antennae) are drawn a bit downward and backward as they are connected to the top of your sternum.

As the inner ends of your clavicles are drawn downward and backward, the outer ends of your clavicles are sent upward and forward.

Since the outer ends of your clavicles are connected to your scapulae (another set of wings), each scapula slides over the back of your rib basket away from your spine and a bit upward.

3. Now bring your sternum forward, allowing the front of you to lengthen.

   As your sternum moves forward your corresponding stretch of spine between your scapulae also moves forward since your ribs connect your sternum and spine.

   This forward movement also opens the front of your rib basket and shoulders.

   The inner ends of your clavicles (butterfly's antennae) are taken forward and upward as they are connected to (and so have to follow) the top of your sternum.

   As the inner ends of your clavicles are sent forward and upward, the outer ends of your clavicles are sent downward and backward.

   As the outer ends of your clavicles are sent downward and backward, each scapula slides over the back of your rib basket toward your spine.

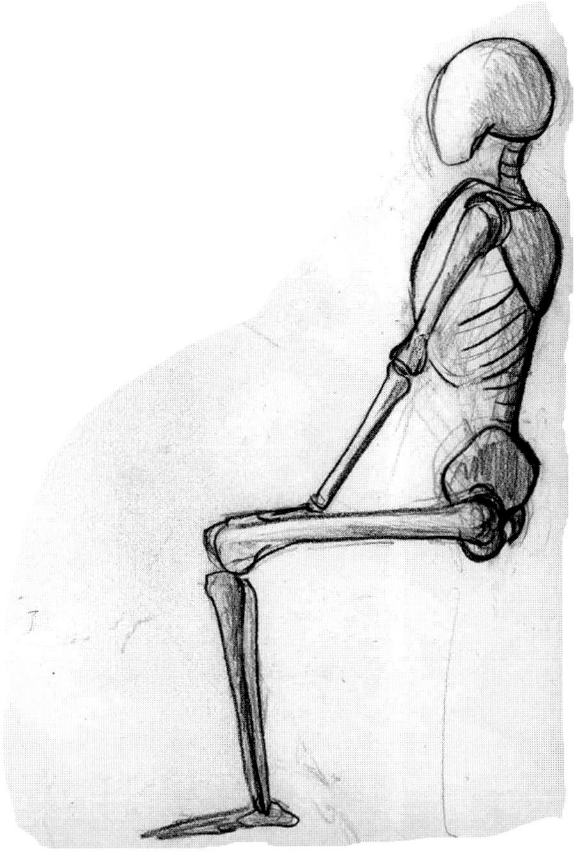

As your stretch of spine between your scapulae is moved backward and forward, allow your whole spine to respond — up to the top of your neck and down to the end of your coccyx (tailbone).

4. Once again, sink your sternum into you causing your thoracic (rib) vertebrae to move backward.
5. Then rearrange your pelvis to rearrange your spine and rib basket (pages 4, 5) to move your sternum and upper thoracic vertebrae forward — so that your scapulae are passively moved toward your spine, sliding over the back of your rib basket.
6. Alternate between your sternum sinking and then your pelvis rearranging your spine and ribs to return your sternum to the horizon — slowly and gently, like a butterfly.

Anytime you catch yourself in a slight slouch, intentionally sink your sternum a little bit more and then let your pelvis rearrange your spine and ribs to "un-sink" your sternum.

This "Butterfly" exercise is a wonderful way to remind your body of its flexibility before you go for a walk. You may also discover that "The Butterfly" can "nip discomfort in the bud" when you have to sit for a long time (e.g. at the computer) or stand for a long time (e.g. at the kitchen sink or at work).

During "The Butterfly," your right and left scapulae mirror each other as they slide away from and toward your spine, with the end result being improved posture. However, to help power your legs while walking or climbing stairs, your scapulae need to alternately slide toward your spine.

The following exercise is inserted here to clarify how your scapulae alternately sliding toward your spine can actually help you walk and climb stairs.

Exercise Nine... "Jog" While Sitting

This is a great rainy day exercise — an alternative to walking outside.

1. Sit on a firm chair that does not have arm rests that could inhibit the movement of your elbows.
2. With your pelvis supporting your posture (page 3), bend your elbows to let them rest against the sides of your body, allowing your shoulders and elbows to give in to gravity (without slouching).

If you allow your elbows to sink a bit lower than your hands your elbows will support your hands! (This is another example of "skeletal engineering.")

The key is to allow your elbows to sink while your pelvis is positioned to lengthen the front of your body.

If you allow your jaw to relax, your elbows will support your hands with even less effort.

Allow the palms of your hands to face each other, as if in relaxed hand-shake position.

3. Slide one scapula (shoulder blade) over your rib basket toward your spine. Then, let that scapula return to its original position. With that same scapula, complete this movement several times.

   Allow the front of both shoulders to be relaxed and open so that your clavicles can allow your scapula to slide.

This is also dynamic positioning for your upper body while aerobic-exercise walking outside.

Notice that each time your scapula slides toward your spine, your elbow is passively taken backward.

Notice that each time your scapula returns to its original position, your elbow is passively moved forward to its original position.

4. Now, each time that scapula slides toward your spine, simultaneously lift the knee on the same side of your body. Do this several times.

   Can you sense how the sliding of your scapula toward your spine initiates a skeletal lever-like process to lift your leg?

5. Alternate between doing #4 and just lifting the knee on that same side of the body without your scapula sliding.

   Can you sense a difference in the amount of effort needed to lift your leg, when you do or don't allow your scapula to slide?

Every time you use your arm, also allow your scapula to move, as the socket of your shoulder ball-and-socket joint is part of your scapula.

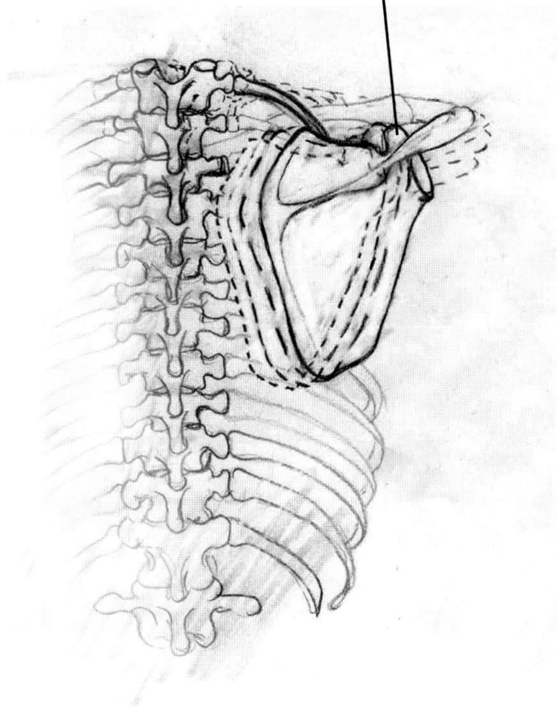

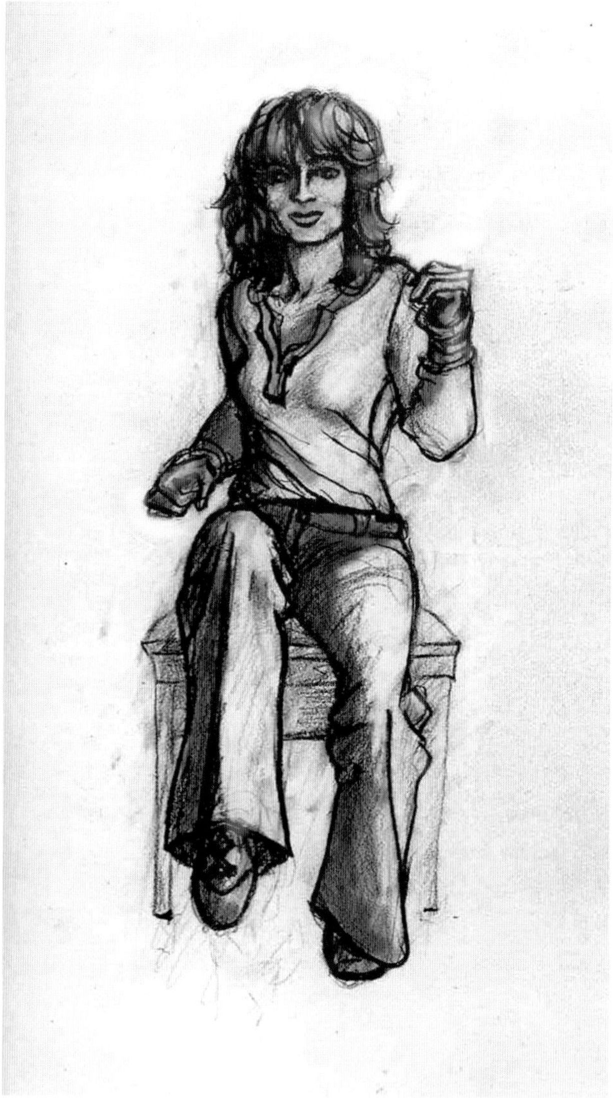

6. With your pelvis supporting your posture so the front of you can lengthen while you're sitting, slide your right scapula toward your spine to lift the right knee and then alternately, your left scapula to lift the left knee.

   As one scapula slides toward your spine, allow the other scapula to passively and simultaneously slide away from your spine!

   To lift your right knee, allow that bony notch at the top of your sternum (jugular notch) to be drawn a bit to the right by your right clavicle and right scapulae.

   To lift your left knee, allow your jugular notch to be drawn a bit to the left by your left clavicle and left scapula.

   You can do this exercise in slow motion as a warm-up for walking or as an aerobic exercise.

   Just make sure you don't hold your breath.

The action of the Sitting Jog can be applied to climbing stairs. This is especially important if there is no handrail as this contra-lateral (scapulae and knees in oppostition) movement provides counterbalance as well as power).

Your shoulders don't have to work hard to help you climb stairs. The key is to allow your scapulae to slide over your rib basket alternately .

- Allow the front of your body to be lengthened, instead of crunched, so that your shoulders can be relaxed in order to be mobile.
- In order to lift your right foot onto the stair above, allow your right scapula to slide toward your spine.

  If you wait until your right foot is already on that stair before you slide your right scapula back you've missed the powerful lever-like process.
- Slide your left scapula toward your spine to initiate the lifting of your left foot onto the next stair above.

Remember, your scapula cannot slide unless your clavicle follows. And, since the inner end of each clavicle is connected to the top of your sternum, allow your rib basket to be pliable so that the bony notch at the top of your sternum also moves.

Instead of trying to "catch up" with the cane, you're going to use its support for push-off.

Your cane can help you have your stride behind you so that your feet and the cane can propel you safely and smoothly forward.

Let's talk about USING A CANE, knowing that it also applies to a walking stick or hiking pole. To simplify, these directions are for the cane being held by the right hand.

(If you hold a cane or walking stick in your left hand, please substitute all "rights" as "lefts.")

Before you start walking, wiggle through your rib basket (page 48) to free up your upper body.

Make sure that the cane held in your right hand is making firm contact with the ground no farther ahead of you than the toes of your left foot.

1. As your right foot moves a bit forward it passes the cane held in your right hand.

   To help your right leg move forward, simultaneously allow your right scapula to slide toward your spine so that your shoulder can stay comfortable as the cane helps to propel you forward.

2. As the cane in your right hand is helping to propel you forward, your

left heel peels off the ground to also propel you forward.

3. Now, as your left foot moves forward, move the cane forward.

   Your right scapula slides away from your spine to enable your shoulder to be comfortable as the cane in your right hand moves forward.

   As your right scapula slides forward, your left scapula is sliding backward to help propel your left leg forward.

4. As your left foot takes its turn to land directly under your body, the cane makes firm contact with the ground parallel with the toes of your left foot.

5. Immediately your left heel (and "the heel" of the cane) begins to peel off the ground to propel your right leg forward so that your right foot can, again, land directly under your body.

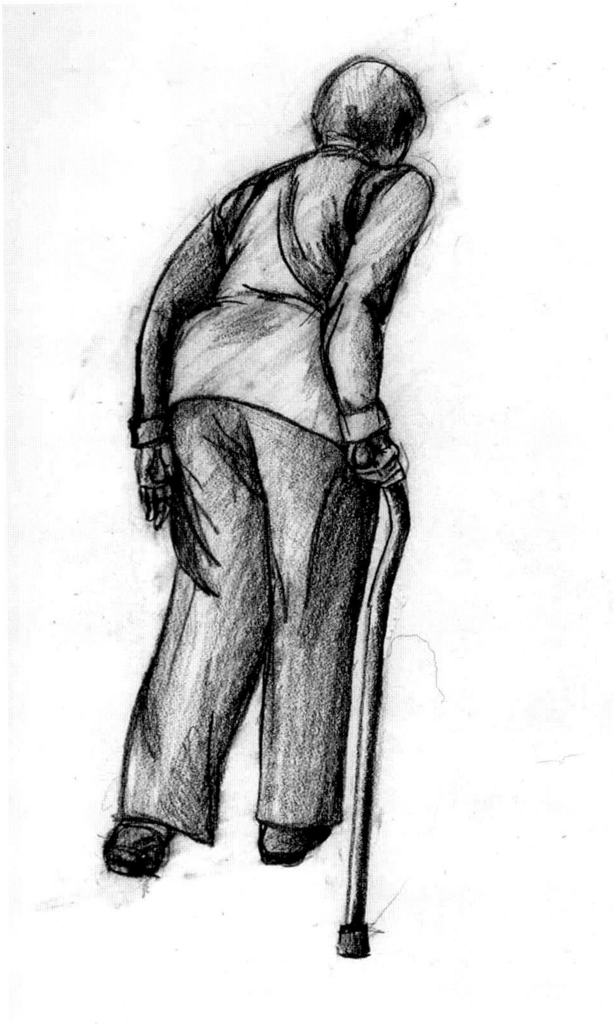

This is contra-lateral walking — your arms (scapulae) and legs (hip joints) moving in opposition.

The human skeleton is "wired" for effortless counter-lateral walking!

There are a lot of details contained in this book. However, once you understand the basics, walking becomes effortless!

Simply allow:

- Your stride to be behind you instead of striding out ahead of yourself;
- Your ankles and feet to be relaxed so you can use the path and the power of each footprint;
- Your torso to be in relaxed lengthening so your sternum is not sunken and your coccyx not tucked;
- Your pelvis to gently rotate to walk your legs while keeping your hip joints healthy;
- Your thorax to be a pliable rib basket so that the rotation of your pelvis travels up your spine to between your scapulae;
- Allow your rib basket to be so relaxed and pliable that your sternum doesn't trap your clavicles and scapulae.
- Your shoulders to be relaxed so that they don't muscularly trap your rib basket and spine, and so that your scapulae can slide to help power your legs.

All of this is what your body was designed to do. You just have to get out of your own way — i.e. relax excessive tension.

SEVENTH STEP…
Walk With Full Awareness

Cut down, or cut out, pain medication before you walk any distance — unless your doctor says you must take your medication on a regular basis. Masking symptoms of pain cheats you from important feedback your body is communicating. Instead pay attention to the pin-pointed reminders your body is giving you.

By making tiny adjustments while you're walking, you'll be able to continue your walk — not give up — with your pain progressively lessening instead of increasing.

If you mask pain, or even if you just ignore pain, you may perpetuate unnecessary wear and tear through your joints.

When your skeleton is well organized, your muscles don't have to exert as much effort to keep you upright or to help you move powerfully.

If your lower back starts hurting:

Have you remembered to allow your stride to be behind you? [See pages 16, 22, 74] Having your stride behind you (with your front foot directly under you instead of out ahead of you) encourages relaxed lengthening instead of crunching.

Are you tightening through your abdominal muscles or lower back, or tucking your coccyx under? [See pages 8–10]

Has stress frozen your rib basket back into a rib "cage" so that the rotation of your walking is happening through your lumbar vertebrae instead of up under your arms? [See pages 47–57]

Is watching the ground drawing your head forward? Remember, your spine is a continuum from the top of your neck down through your pelvis. How you position one portion of your spine affects your whole spine.

To prevent back problems, allow any movement — whether walking or reaching — to flow the entire length of your spine.

If your hip starts hurting:

Have you remembered to allow your stride to be behind you? [See pages 16, 18]

Are you irritating your hip ball-and-socket joint by preventing the socket (part of your pelvis) from moving with the ball (part of your leg)? [See pages 45, 74, 95]

Have you remembered to allow the front of your body to lengthen instead of crunching your abs, tightening through your lower back, or tucking your coccyx under? [See pages 8–10]

Has your chest frozen into a rib "cage" preventing your pelvis from rotating as you walk? [See pages 49–50]

Are you powering your arms so hard that your hips follow your shoulders instead of your pelvis rotating opposite your shoulders? If so, each hip is rotating back right at the moment it needs to rotate forward and vice versa. [See pages 61–62]

If your knees start hurting:

Have you remembered to allow your stride to be behind you? [See page 34] Having your stride behind you, instead of out ahead of you, allows your knees to be securely supported every step of the way.

Have your knees gone into hyperextension (actually bent backward a bit from neutral)? [See pages 13, 18]

Has your pelvis stopped rotating so it isn't helping your legs walk? [See pages 46, 57-58]

Has your chest frozen back into a rib "cage" so that your pelvis can't (for the moment) walk your legs? [See pages 49-50]

Have you remembered to have your footprints fully support your knees while walking? [See pages 24, 32, 35-43]

Have you tightened through your ankles or toes? [See pages 27-29]

Have you remembered to allow space between your 1st and 2nd toes and the 4th and 5th toes so that your middle three toes support your knee? [See pages 25, 32]

If your heels are tender:

Have you remembered to allow your stride to be behind you? [See page 18] Striding out ahead of yourself is a sure way to pound your heels into the ground.

Have you remembered to allow your ankles and feet to be relaxed and flexible so that each heel can easily peel off the ground? [See pages 31-32]

Make sure you're not hyper-extending your knees, as that forces your heels into the ground.

If the "ball" of a foot becomes tender:

Have you remembered to allow your toes to relax? Pulling your toes upward forces the heads of the metatarsals downward into the ground.

Are your shoes or boots squeezing the spaces between the length of your toes? [See pages 25, 32, 39]

Make sure that you're not subconsciously pushing the ball of your foot into the floor or a rung of your chair when you're concentrating on paper work, a musical instrument, or your computer.

When you use your footprints the way nature intended, you even out the distribution of labor so no one part of your foot is forced into the ground.

If your neck becomes uncomfortable:

Are you looking down at your feet as you walk? Instead, trust the path of your footprints [see page 36-40] so that you can look ahead of you to anticipate the cracks in the sidewalk, tree roots, or bicyclist headed your way.

Have you remembered to allow your pelvis to support your posture? If not, your chest may be sunken and the neck-end of your spine can't relax because your head is forward? [See pages 3-8, 65-66]

Are you tightening through your lower back, glutes, or along your coccyx? Any of those three flattens your lumbar curve, which moves your head forward enough to cause strain through your neck.

Is there rigidity in that stretch of spine directly below your neck, between your scapulae? If so, wiggle through your rib basket. [See pages 48, 63-66]

If your shoulders, arms, or hands become uncomfortable:

Are you trying to maintain upright posture by pulling your shoulders back? Instead allow your pelvis to support your posture. [See pages 2–5]

Have you remembered to allow your clavicles to allow your scapulae to alternately slide toward and away from your spine? [See pages 59, 67–70, 73]

Have you remembered to allow your rib basket to be freely pliable so that your jugular notch allows your clavicles to allow your scapulae to alternate sliding toward and away from your spine? [See pages 48, 70–75, 109]

Have you remembered to allow your elbows to give in to gravity to support your lower arms and hands? [See page 68]

Are the palms of your hands facing the ground, the sky, straight ahead of you, or facing behind you? Instead, allow your hands to relax into a hand-shake position, i.e. your thumbs forward or toward the sky. [See page 93]

If your bunion is painful, or becoming larger:

Have you remembered to allow space between your 1st and 2nd toes and the 4th and 5th toe? [See pages 25, 31-32]

You can wrap your second toe with lambs wool or buy spacers to insert between your big toe and second toe to encourage your big toe not to angle toward your second toe.

Have you remembered to allow the length of your 4th metatarsal to lever you onto the ball of your foot instead of jaywalking across your foot to the bunion? [See pages 25-26]

The adjustments you make as a result of all this awareness are exactly what will make your walking more powerful as well as more comfortable.

EIGHTH STEP…
Walking As Exercise

We need to walk — not just to move from one spot to another, but also to maintain muscle and bone integrity. The largest bones in the body, as well as the largest muscles, are below the waist. You can use the gravitational pull that we all live in to strengthen those large bones and all the vertebrae through your spine with every step that you take.

You don't have to work hard to get a good workout when you allow your skeletal connections to cooperate!

We all need weight-bearing exercise. Without gravity, astronauts in prime condition can lose bone density during less than a week while weightless out in space.

WARM-UPS...

Save your stretches for after you've exercised when your muscles are well warmed and your joints are well lubed.

These warm-ups are all about freeing your body for flexible, efficient, pleasurable mobility.

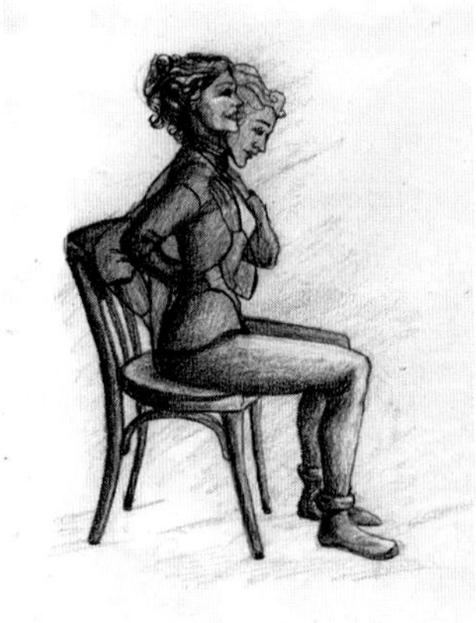

The Butterfly (page 63) reminds your upper body and your whole spine to be available for powerful, comfortable walking.

This exercise also helps you regain flexibility through that stretch of spine between your shoulder blades which can become stuck so easily.

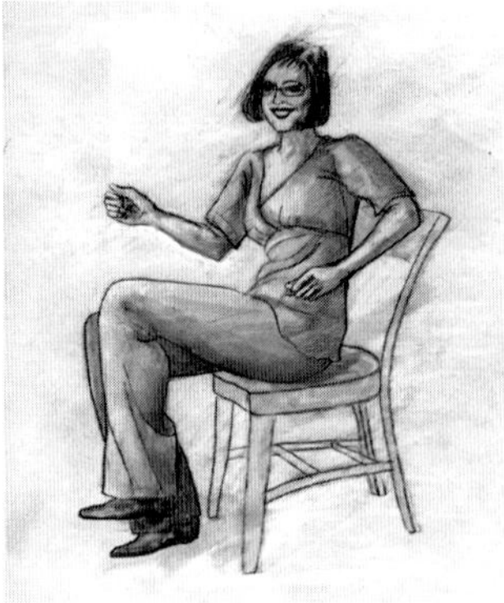

"Jog" While Sitting (page 67) reminds you to allow your upper body to help you walk.

This is a great rainy day alternative to walking outside.

EXERCISE TEN...
Rotate Pelvis to "Walk" Your Knees While Sitting

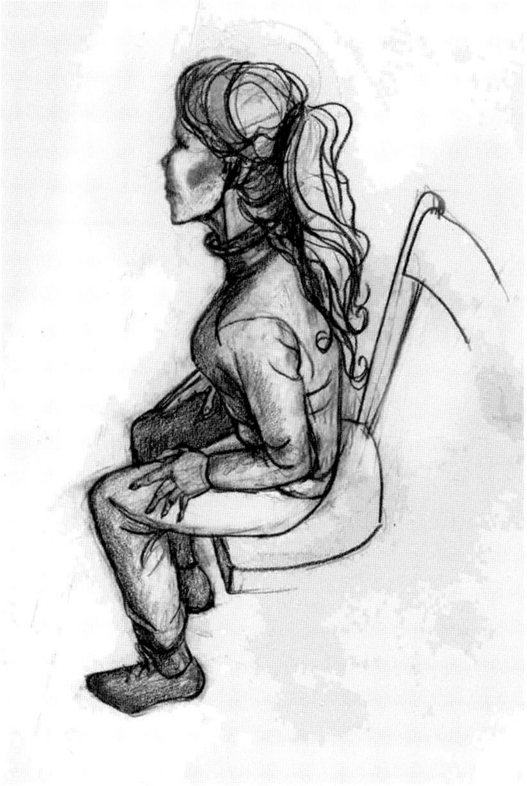

1. Sit on a firm chair or bench with your pelvis supporitng your posture (page 5).

2. Place your feet a comfortable distance apart and parallel to each other. It's important that your feet stay in place (not lift or slide) throughout this exercise.

3. Rotate your pelvis so that one hip joint travels a bit backward and, because your pelvis is a bowl, the other hip joint travels a bit forward simultaneously.

   Notice what happens to the knee of the leg connected through the hip joint that moved forward. Did it passively lengthen away from you?

   Notice what happens to the knee of the leg connected through the hip joint that moved backward. Has it passively been drawn backward a bit?

4. With your knees remaining parallel (straight ahead as if on parallel tracks) and your feet staying in place (not sliding), slowly rotate your pelvis left and right.

   As your left hip joint rides back, your right hip joint rides forward and your right knee lengthens/"walks" forward.

   As your right hip joint rides back, your left hip joint rides forward and your left knee lengthens/"walks" forward.

Allow this rotation of your pelvis to travel up your spine to between your scapulae.

5. Allow your rib basket to follow the rotation of your pelvis, resulting in movement up under your scapulae (shoulder blades) and up under your arms.

6. Rotate your pelvis right and left a little bit quicker and even more gently — the faster the rotation, the tinier the movement.

   Allow your head "to float" so that the movement can travel up your spine through your neck.

The faster you move, the more you need to move your body gently — your body gliding instead of roaring.

EXERCISE ELEVEN... Flexible Feet & Ankles, Scapulae Freed

1. Stand with your feet parallel and with your pelvis supporting your posture (page 5).

2. Peel one heel off the ground and then, as that heel returns to the ground, peel the other heel away from the ground.

   Both feet remain in place with the ball of each foot keeping contact with the ground.

   Allow each knee, in turn, to bend and move forward as the heel peels off the ground.

   Make sure that neither knee goes into hyperextension (locked backward) when the heel takes its turn to be solid on the ground.

3. Allow your ankles to relax as you continue alternately peeling one heel off the ground and then the other.

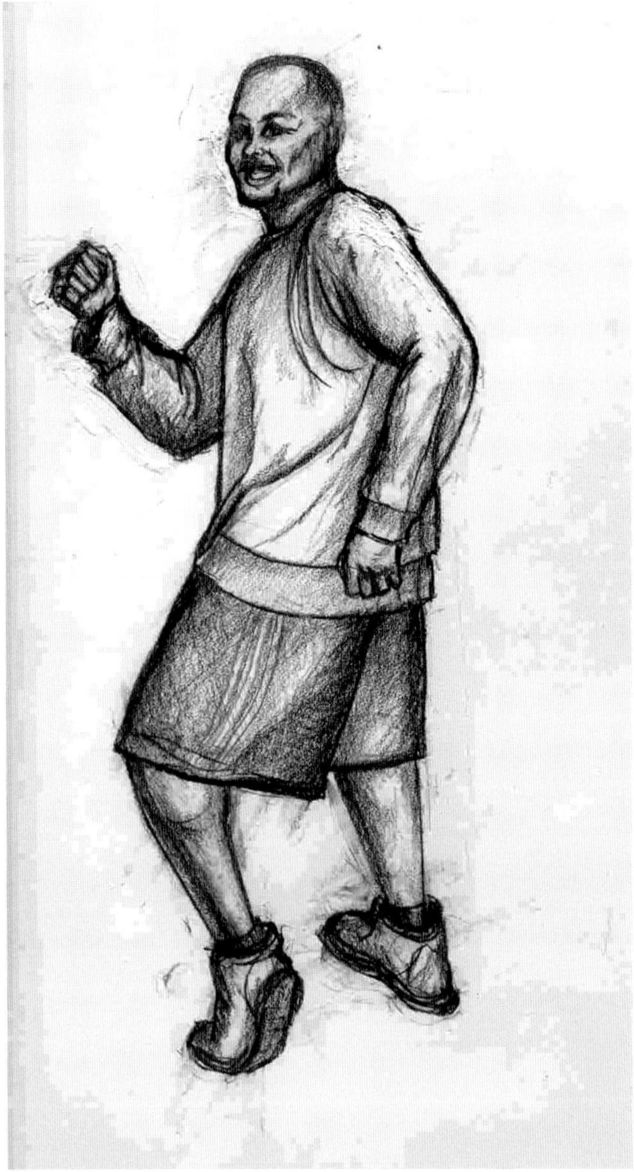

Allow the front of each ankle to lengthen as its heel peels away from the ground.

Allow the back of each ankle to fold as the front of that ankle lengthens.

4. Allow your rib basket to allow your pelvis to rotate as your heels alternately peel off the ground.

   As your left heel peels off the ground, allow your pelvis to rotate to the right so that your left hip is more forward than your right hip.

   As your right heel peels off the ground, allow your pelvis to rotate to the left so that your right hip is more forward than your left hip.

5. With your feet remaining in place, allow the rotation of your pelvis to initiate the peeling of your heels off the ground. (This is moving proximally instead of distally.)

   As your left hip is rotated forward, notice that your left knee is moved forward which peels your left heel off the ground.

   As your right hip is rotated forward, notice that your right knee is moved forward which peels your right heel off the ground.

6. Eventually allow the rotation of your pelvis to alternately peel your heels off the ground, moving first one femur (upper leg bone) forward and then the other. Your feet remain in place.

   Each time your left hip is moved forward to peel your left heel off the ground, allow the front of your left shoulder to open so that your left scapula can slide toward your spine.

   Each time your right hip is moved forward to peel your right heel off the ground, allow the front of your right shoulder to open so that your right scapula can slide toward your spine.

Now you're walking in place — the perfect warm-up for exercise walking.

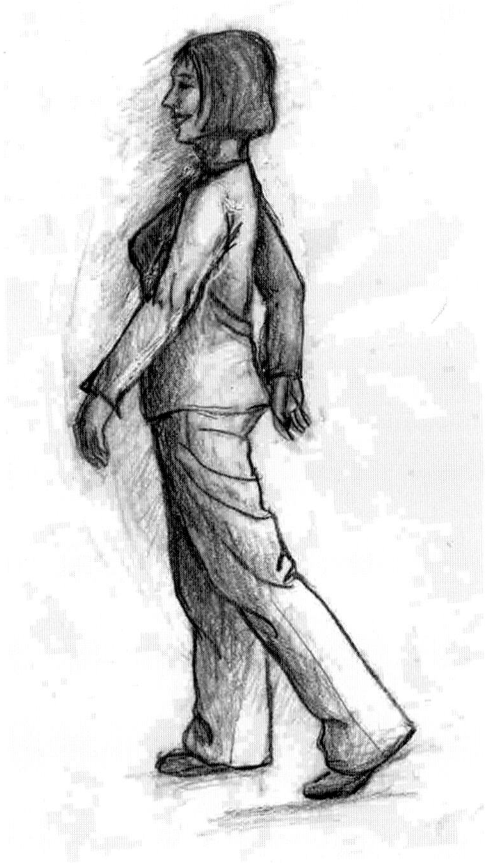

WALKING IN THE MALL OR PARK...

Apply STEPS ONE through SEVEN in this book — plus:

Breathe!!!! Do not hold your breath!

Breath-holding can become so habitual that it's below one's level of awareness.

Breath-holding can be the cause for unnecessary fatigue.

If you're holding your breath, you're not allowing your rib basket the pliability your body needs for comfortable, powerful walking.

Interval Walking

To build your stamina you can alternate between slower walking and faster walking.

While walking slower, allow your arms to be down by your sides.

While walking faster, bend your elbows and let them sink into gravity so that your hands are supported by your bent elbows.

In either case, allow your jaw to relax.

If you want to walk faster — instead of making your legs work harder, allow your scapulae to slide more freely.

In either case, allow your shoulders to be relaxed so that the front of you can lengthen and your scapulae can move freely to help your lower body walk.

In either case, allow your hands to be in a relaxed hand-shake position, i.e. when your arms are down by your sides, your thumbs will face forward, and when your elbows are bent, your thumbs will face toward the sky. (Don't tense your thumbs.)

Even if you have a purse hanging from your shoulder, your rib basket and clavicles (collarbones) can allow your scapulae to slide alternately toward your spine to help propel your legs.

In either case, of course, allow your stride to be behind you (pages 16, 18, and 34) instead of stepping out ahead of yourself.

Walking with a Wheeled Walker

Even if you don't need to use a walker all of the time, your walker can remind you to incorporate good body dynamics as you safely exercise.

Briefly experiment to confirm that stepping far out in front of yourself is absolutely unnecessary:

Notice if you press downward into the walker and grip it more firmly when your stride is out ahead of you.

Notice that when your stride is behind you, your hands and arms are just the connecting link between you and the walker.

- Wiggle through your rib basket to remind yourself to relax. [See page 48]
- Allow your ankles and toes to be relaxed so nothing interferes with each heel taking its turn to peel off the ground.

- Allow your shoulders to be relaxed so that they don't prevent movement through your rib basket and spine.
- Your hips and spine are safer when you allow your pelvis to rotate a little bit — not making it happen, but allowing it to happen.

  Allow your sacrum (therefore your whole pelvis) to rotate a bit around to the right to take your left hip joint forward to move your left leg forward and, simultaneously, your right hip joint backward to help the right heel take its turn to peel off the ground behind you.

  Allow your pelvis to rotate a bit around to the left to take your right hip joint forward to move your right leg forward and, simultaneously, your left hip joint and left leg backward.

  Allow this rotation to travel up into your rib basket up under your arms.

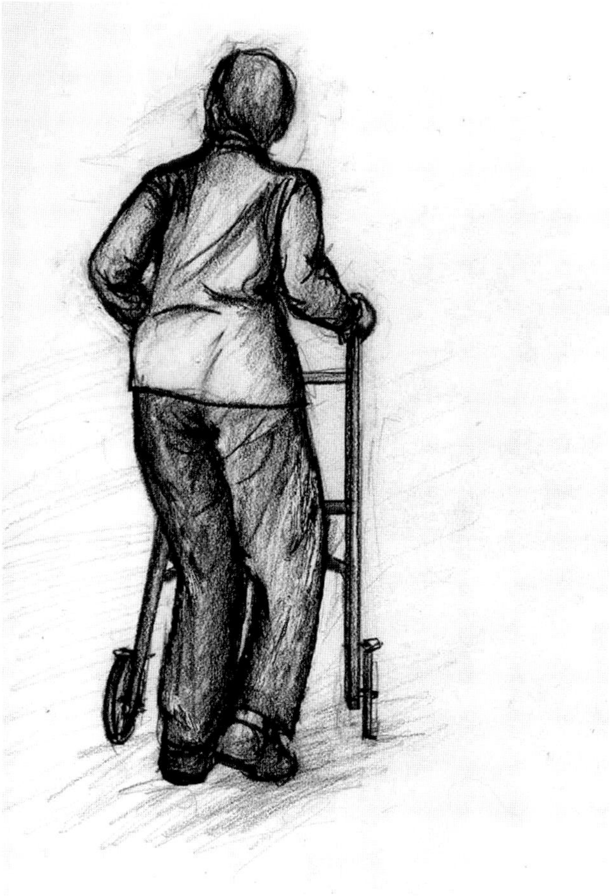

COOL-DOWNS...

Warm up and cool down even if you're not going for a long hike.

Even after exercising, you want to ease into stretching. As of yet, it's not easy to replace ligaments even though the science of hip and knee replacements is being perfected. The purpose of your ligaments is to keep your joints safely in place as you move. If you continually overstretch a ligament, it loses its elasticity.

To use a metaphor, if you continually stretch a rubber band to its max, it wears out, losing its capability to snugly hold something in place. (Think about this the next time someone suggests that you should pull your foot back toward your buttocks — as this causes overstretching through the ligaments that hold your knee in place.)

The metaphor of a rubber band also applies to the scenario of stretching hard during the stage before elasticity is worn out — it pops back as soon as the stretch lets up. The medical name for this "rubber band" reflex is "myotatic."

Linger Walking

As you near the end of your walk, begin your cool-down by walking slower. (You know it's not a good idea to walk fast all the way to your car or front door and then sit for a half hour.) When your car or home is within your sight, allow each foot to linger just a split second longer:

> Linger (pause briefly) right at the moment each foot takes its turn for the heel to peel off the ground behind you. This creates a gentle stretch through the front of each ankle and encourages lengthening through the front of your spine and the front of your whole body.
>
> Make sure your stride is underneath and behind you (see pages 16, 18, 32) all the time — but especially during this Linger Walking.

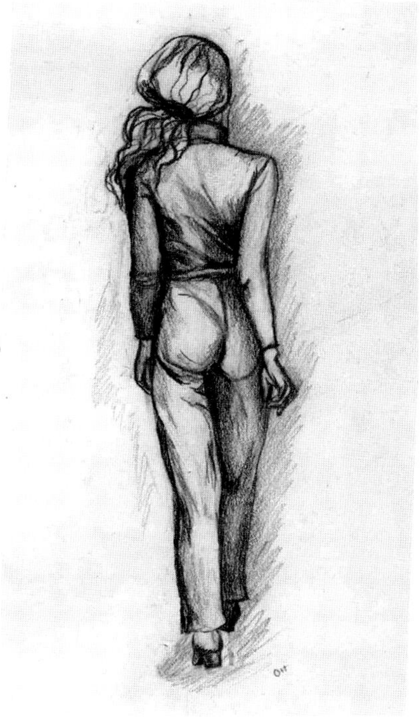

Exercise Twelve... Walking Backward

Walking backward is therapeutic for your knees, hips, and spine as well as a perfect cool-down after any exercise. Just make sure you are in a location in which it's safe to walk backward — i.e. no stairs nearby, no one close by that you could collide into, and no cars or bicycles that could collide into you.

1. Look over your shoulder to make sure it's safe to walk backward.

2. "Sit" your pelvis back a bit so that you bend just a little bit more through your hip joints, your sternum (breastbone) facing the horizon. (You could use the image of buoyant water supporting this position.)

3. Lead with your sacrum (the base of your spine in the center back of your pelvis) as if a magnet is drawing you backward.

   Allow your feet to simply follow. You defeat the purpose if you carefully place your feet behind you or try to lead backward with your feet.

If you ever sense you're losing your balance, immediately release your coccyx (tailbone) backward as if to sit down. This accordion pleating (folding through the hip joints, knees, and ankles) is what most people automatically do when waves rock a boat.

4. Walk forward a few steps.

5. Double check that it's safe to walk backward again.

6. "Sit" your pelvis again and allow your sacrum to draw you backward with your feet simply following instead of leading.

Exercise Thirteen... Standing Inch Worm

This exercise is more than simply a cool-down. This useful technique will help make your back more comfortable any time, any place, while providing a gentle hamstring stretch.

1. Stand facing some solid surface that is approximately waist-high (possibilities include countertop, fence, fender of your car, or back of a park bench).

2. Position your feet parallel to each other, a comfortable distance apart and approximately 10-12 inches from that solid object (close enough that your elbows are bent at about a 90 degree angle while you're in

The hamstring stretch in this and the next exercise is going to be in the forward leg. This stretch through your leg and your spine is directly related to your sternum (breastbone) facing the horizon.

upright posture with your fingertips resting on that solid surface).

3. Slide one foot backward until the toes of that foot are opposite the heel of your other foot. (At this point the full footprint of each foot is making contact with the ground.)

Do not sink your chest or tuck your coccyx (tailbone) at any time throughout this exercise.

4. With your fingertips resting on that surface, allow the front of you to lengthen so that your sternum can face out to the horizon while your shoulders and elbows give in to gravity. As you do this lengthening through the front of you, allow the heel of the foot that is back a bit to peel off the ground.

5. With your sternum facing out to the horizon, lower yourself a little bit by bending through your hip joints and knees. Your heel will return to the ground.

6. With your sternum still facing toward the horizon, have your coccyx (tailbone) draw you backward so that you bend even more through your hip joints.

This backward movement will draw the toes of whichever foot is forward a little bit away from the ground. Allow this to happen, don't make it happen.

Allow your sternum to remain facing the horizon instead of downward. Do not round your spine into a slouch.

The combination of your sternum not dropping downward while your coccyx draws your spine backward creates a gentle yet effective hamstring stretch through the leg that is forward — i.e. if you let your sternum sink you won't get the hamstring stretch.

7. Now, allow your pelvis to return to the original position so that your pelvis can once again support your posture.

   As your pelvis moves your spine forward and upward and the front of you lengthens, the toes of your front foot return to the ground and the heel of the foot that is back will leave the ground.

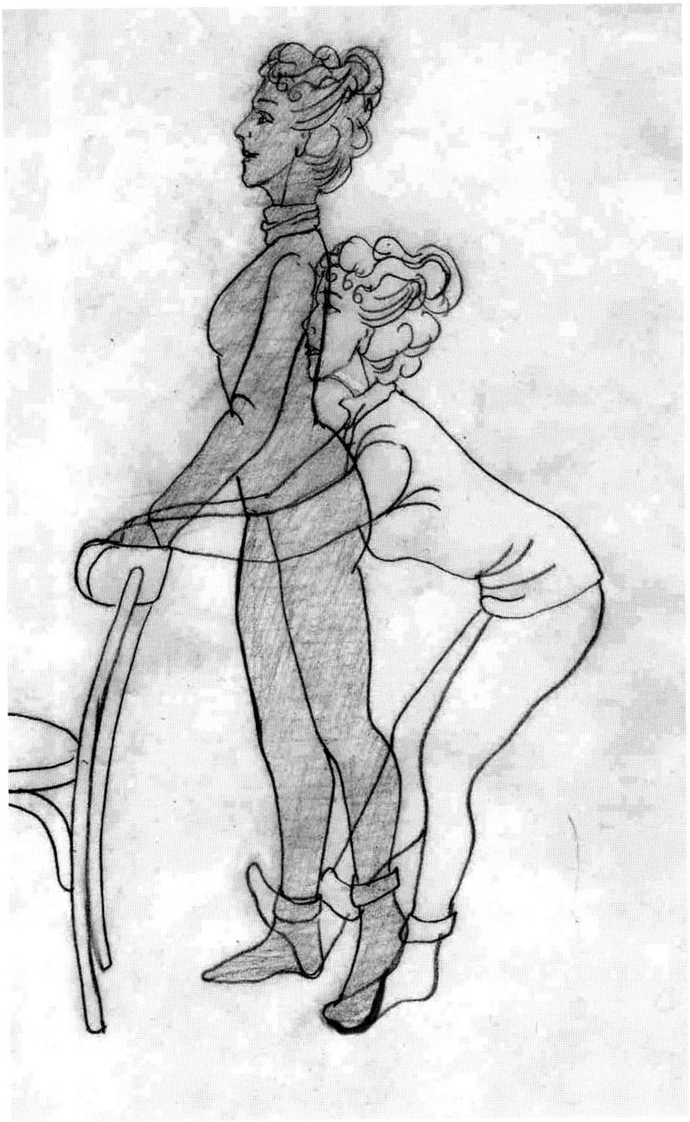

You want the bending that is required for this (and the next) exercise to happen through your hip joints, not your spine.

8. Slowly repeat the sequence of #5, #6, and #7 a number of times. Your feet remain in place throughout — it is rocking on your feet, not sliding your feet.

   The toes of the front foot are drawn away from the ground a little bit as your body is drawn backward.

   As your body moves forward, those toes settle onto the ground and the heel of the back foot is drawn away from the ground
9. Switch the position of your feet so your other leg can take its turn to receive this gentle stretch.
10. With your feet in their new positions slowly repeat the sequence of #5, #6, and #7.

Exercise Fourteen... Foot on curb, stair, or car bumper

This exercise also stretches hamstrings while relaxing your back and joints. Again, the position of your sternum and your coccyx are directly related to the degree of hamstring stretch you'll receive.

1. Stand about a foot (more if you're very tall) from a curb or bottom stair — far enough away from that object so that one leg would be slightly bent if you put the ball of that foot on the curb or bottom stair.

   If you're outside and that object is a curb, please make sure that you are not vulnerable to a car pulling into your space.

2. Place the "ball" of one foot on that curb or bottom stair, making sure that neither foot is angled. The other foot is directly under your body.

You want the toes of the foot that is up and the foot that is under you to be facing forward so that each knee is fully supported.

Allow all of your toes to relax so that the middle three toes of each foot can support each knee.

Fold through your hip joints so that your coccyx (tailbone) is not tucked under you.

This lifting of the sternum is what gives you the hamstring stretch — and the lifting of the sternum is possible only if your coccyx is not tucked under you.

3. Lift your sternum (breastbone) to face the horizon.

4. Hold that position for a slow count of ten or more — don't bounce, just hold the stretch.

   If you want more of a stretch: Instead of taking your knee farther forward, release your coccyx a little farther backward while lifting your sternum a bit more (the opposite of rounding into a slouch).

5. When you're ready, switch the position of your legs.

   One foot is directly underneath you and the ball of the other foot is on the curb or bottom stair.

   Make sure that you fold through your hip joints with your sternum facing the horizon, not the ground.

6. If you want even more of a stretch put your foot on the second stair or on your car bumper.

   Hold the position, don't bounce. Make sure that your coccyx is released and that your sternum is facing the horizon.

   If you want yet another degree of stretch — instead of making the knee of the foot that is on the car bumper go farther away from you, simply take your coccyx back a bit farther while your sternum remains facing the horizon.

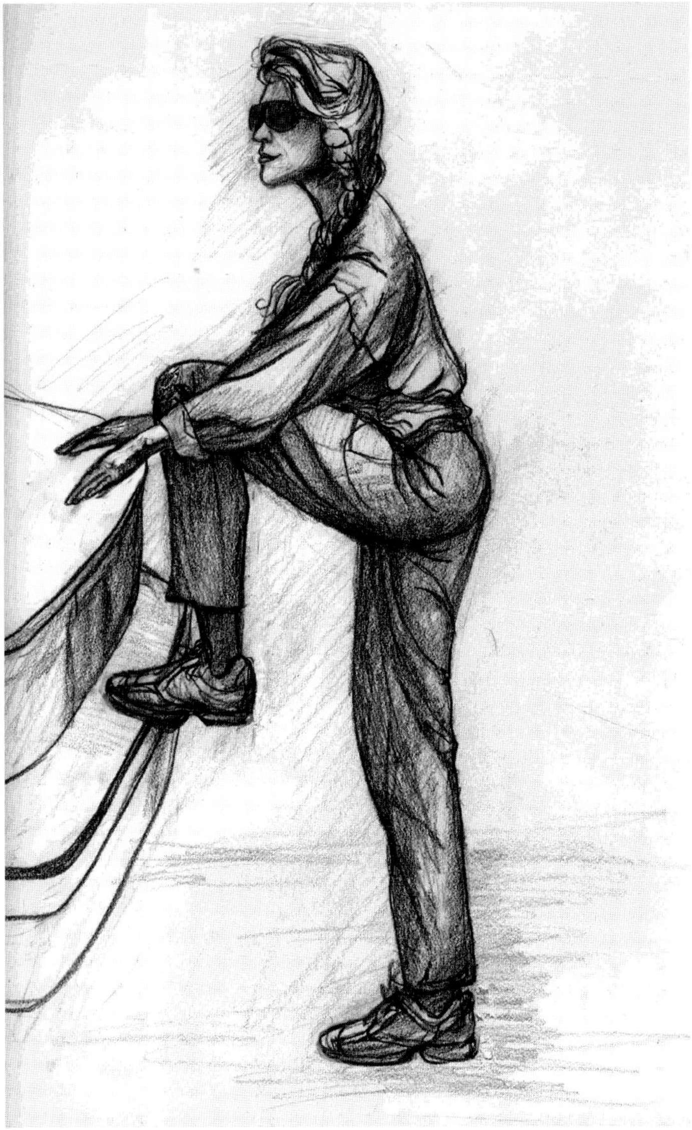

Distance Hiking…

If you're serious about hiking, you've probably read this whole book with great interest — if you just skipped to this section please go back to understand the groundwork details.

- Rough terrain will not be as much of an issue if, in preparation for your hike, you enhance the flexibility of your ankles and feet (pages 87-89) and the pliability of your rib basket (page 48).
- Especially if you're wearing a backpack, instead of striding out ahead of your body, have your stride under and behind you.

  It's the heel of the foot that is taking its turn peeling off the ground behind you that powers you forward.

  As one foot is behind you, the other foot is directly under your body fully supporting you and your backpack!

- With every step, allow some space between the 1st (big) toe and the 2nd toe, and also between the 5th (little) toe and 4th toe, so that your middle three toes of each foot can support each kneecap.
- Make sure that you don't "jaywalk" from the heel to the base of the 1st toe (bunion territory). The 4th metatarsal of each foot can smoothly lever you onto the "ball" of your foot as your heel peels off the ground.
- Make sure your shoes or boots allow bend-ability through the "ball" of each foot.
- Make sure that your foot doesn't slide forward in your shoe or boot on the downhill. In addition to having a good fit, you could insert flexible pads.
- **Never, ever hyperextend your knees.**

Even if you're wearing a backpack, the top of your sternum and your clavicles can rotate a bit to help walk your legs.

- Breathe into your back to relax your back — especially if you're wearing a backpack. (Your lungs are like balloons that can expand out to the sides and backward as well as forward.)

  This does not mean hyperventilate — it simply means to breathe the way nature intended. Breathing shallowly and endurance are antithetical.

- Allow your head "to float" (like a helium-filled balloon) to relax muscular tension through your neck and shoulders, allowing your spine to rotate up under your skull.

  You want to be able to look ahead, or around yourself, independent of the rotation of your shoulders.

- Make sure that your hips are supporting the backpack, so that your clavicles and scapulae can rotate subtly in spite of the shoulder straps.

Imagine that you have a tiny penlight nestled in the bony notch directly beneath your throat (jugular notch formed by the top of your sternum and the inner ends of your clavicles).

Allow that imaginary penlight to rotate to the right to help bring your right leg forward to be underneath you as, simultaneously, your left heel peels off the ground behind you.

Allow that imaginery penlight to rotate to the left to help bring your left leg forward to be underneath you as, simultaneously, your right heel peels off the ground behind you.

- You could explore the advantages of trekking with two hiking poles:

The idea is not to put them out ahead of yourself (pulling yourself toward them), but using each one, in turn, for push-off matched with the opposite foot.

Let's think in terms of two hiking poles with each pole having its own footprint.

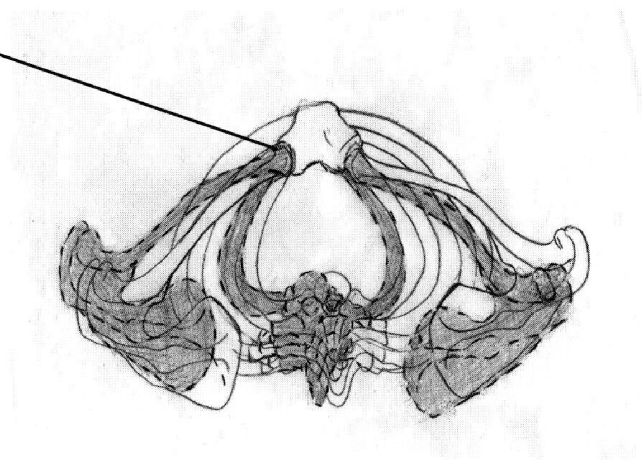

Allow the propulsion from each heel peeling off the ground to travel through your spine up under your skull and through your rib basket to the top of your sternum,

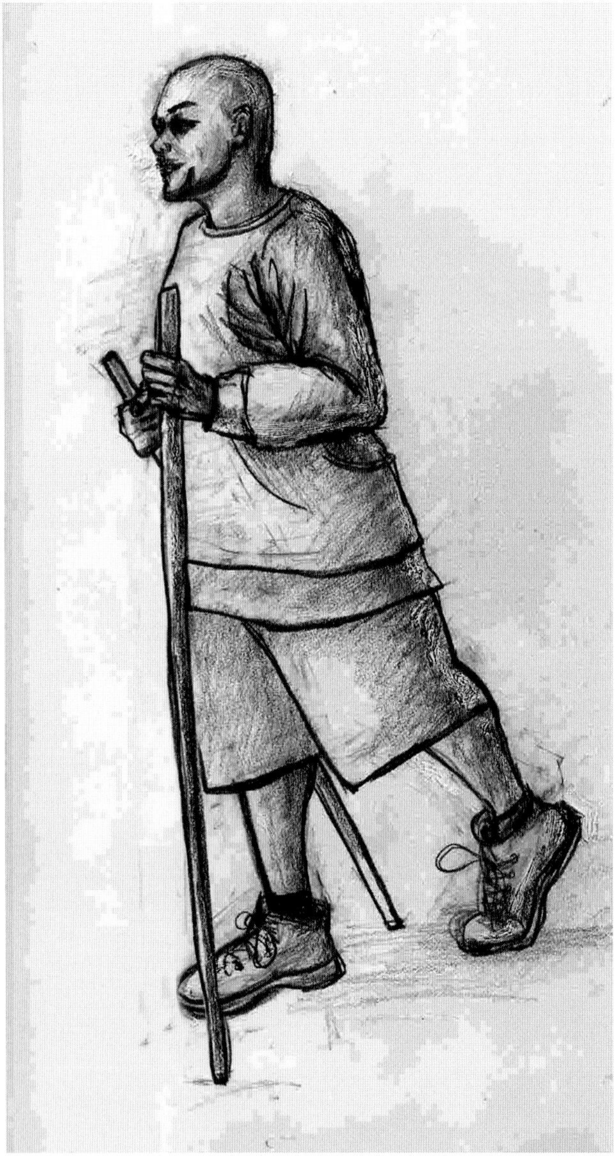

For two hiking poles:

1. When your right foot is momentarily taking its turn to be directly underneath you, supporting you and your backpack with its full footprint, the full footprint of the hiking pole in your left hand makes firm contact with the ground parallel to the toe of your right shoe.

   Simultaneously, as your left heel takes its turn to peel off the ground behind you to propel you forward, the "heel" of the hiking pole in your right hand also peels a bit off of the ground to help propel you forward.

2. When your left foot is momentarily taking its turn to be directly underneath you, supporting you and your backpack with its full footprint, the full footprint of the hiking pole in your right hand makes firm contact with the ground parallel to the toe of your left shoe.

Simultaneously, as your right heel takes its turn to peel off the ground behind you to propel you forward, the "heel" of the hiking pole in your left hand also peels a bit off the ground to help propel you forward.

3. Allow the bony notch directly beneath your throat to gently rotate a tiny bit side-to-side so your clavicles and scapulae slide to keep your shoulders comfortable as you use your hiking poles to power yourself forward.

   Allow that imaginary penlight in your jugular notch "to shine" a little bit to the right to help your right leg move underneath you to support you and your backpack and "to shine" to the left to help your left leg move underneath you, taking its turn to support you and your backpack.

   As your jugular notch subtly rotates, your clavicles will rotate and your scapulae will alternately slide over your rib basket toward your spine.

Remember the socket of your shoulder ball-and-socket joint is part of your scapula (shoulder blade). If you don't move the socket as well as the ball of each shoulder joint, you are setting yourself up for joint pain as well as loss of power.

The roadmap for healthful movement is in your skeleton.

This gentle sliding of each scapula powers the leg on that side of your body forward. So, don't force your scapulae or you'll end up kicking out ahead of yourself instead of having your stride behind you.

To summarize, as the heel of your left foot is peeling off the ground behind you to power you forward, simultaneously allow your jugular notch to rotate a tiny bit to the right so your right scapula slides toward your spine, taking your right elbow backward so that the cane in your right hand can also power you forward.

One clear day my hiking partner and I rode a ski lift up to a beautiful lookout point "just to have a picnic lunch with a view." As we eyed a trail that traversed the mountain in the direction of an interesting town, we decided to head out. Since I didn't have my hiking poles with me for this spur-of-the-moment, long-distance adventure, I pretended to have a hiking pole in each hand to encourage my upper body to help walk my legs. The results of this experiment were excellent — highly recommended.

- Make your rest breaks even more beneficial with skeletal awareness.

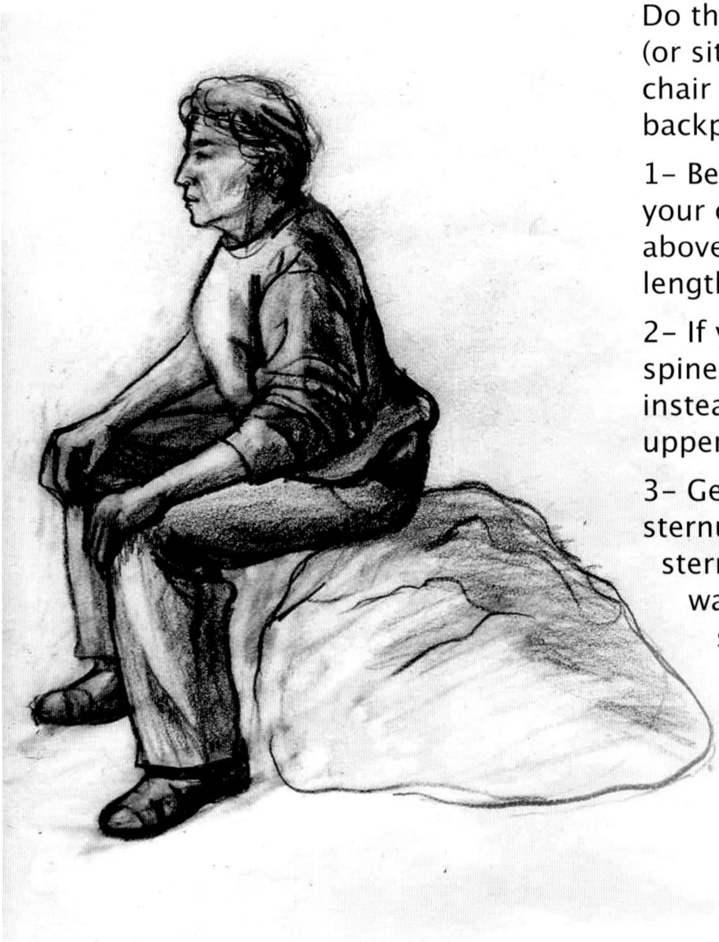

Do the following stretch while standing (or sitting on some object about chair height), preferably without your backpack on:

1- Bend through your hip joints with your coccyx released, your hands just above your knees, and your spine lengthened (not rounded in a slouch).

2- If you want just a bit more of a spine-stretch, rest your forearms instead of your hands on your upper legs.

3- Gently, alternately sink your sternum into you and then lift your sternum forward and up to gently wake up movement through the stretch of spine between your scapulae (shoulder blades).

- Before you return your pack to your back, wiggle through your ribs (page 48):

  To free up your hips and spine so that your pelvis can support your posture;

  To remind you that your jugular notch, clavicles, and scapulae need to be mobile;

  To remind you not to tighten through your abs or gluts — so that your pelvis can support your posture and your backpack;

  And to allow your pelvis to be free to rotate a bit to help walk your legs.

- Before you resume your hike, alternate one heel then the other peeling off the ground in place (page 87), reminding your ankles and feet to be relaxed as you walk with your stride behind you.

- Be sure you cool down before you sit for a long time in your vehicle or around a campfire. All of the cool-downs already taught (pages 94-103) are even more important after a day of hiking!

Before you head out on any trail, be sure you're clear about your inner road map (your skeletal connections) and your inner compass (skeletal engineering).

About the author and the Feldenkrais Method® of Somatic Education

As an exercise trainer for those with physical challenges and a Guild Certified Feldenkrais Practitioner^cm, Pamela Kihm motivates people to choose more healthful movement options. All of Pamela's books in the PainFreeChoices® series are based on the Feldenkrais Method® of Somatic Education developed by Moshe Feldenkrais DSc.

With degrees in engineering as well as physics, Dr. Feldenkrais (1904–1984) was a genius at understanding and teaching biomechanics—"skeletal engineering" — e.g. when your skeleton is well organized, your muscles don't have to exert as much effort to keep you upright and to help you move powerfully.

"We make the impossible possible, the possible easy, and the easy elegant."

—Moshe Feldenkrais

For more information about the *Feldenkrais Method of Somatic Education* and to locate a *Guild Certified Feldenkrais Practitioner^cm* near you, contact the *Feldenkrais Guild® of North America* through www.feldenkrais.com

Resources for books, CDs, and DVDs based on the Feldenkrais Method® of Somatic Education include:

www.feldenkraisguild.com/bookstore

www.feldenkraisresources.com

www.achievingexcellence.com

SUBJECT INDEX

EXERCISE INDEX